Healing Archetypes and Symbols

STEWART A. SWERDLOW

and

JANET DIANE MOURGLIA-SWERDLOW

Expansions Publishing Company, Inc.
Saint Joseph, Michigan
USA

HEALING ARCHETYPES AND SYMBOLS

Published by: Expansions Publishing Company, Inc.
P.O. Box 12
Saint Joseph, Michigan 49085 USA
269-519-8036
Skype: eventsatexpansions
customersupport@expansions.com
www.expansions.com

ISBN: 978-0-9740144-7-0

Cover Design: Alison Hilary Corbalis
www.alisoncorbalis.blogspot.com

Without action, the words are powerless.
Action is actually archetype in motion.

The information provided in this publication is not an attempt to practice medicine or provide specific medical advice, nor is it a substitute for medical care.

We always recommend consulting with a healthcare professional before starting any diet, exercise, supplementation, or medication program.

You assume full responsibility for using any information provided and agree that we are not responsible or liable for any claim resulting from its use by you or any user.

To Patricia Lynn O'Bryant

Thank you for the many years of dedication, service, loyalty and unconditional love. You have stayed by our side through every possible event. You are unique among humans. We are grateful that you are a part of our lives.

Books by Stewart A. Swerdlow & Janet Diane Mourglia-Swerdlow

Blue Blood, True Blood: Conflict & Creation

Decoding Your Life: An Experiential Course in Self-Reintegration

Healer's Handbook: A Journey Into Hyperspace

Healing Archetypes and Symbols

Hyperspace Helper

Hyperspace Plus

Montauk: Alien Connection

Stewart Says…

True Reality of Sexuality

True World History: Humanity's Saga

White Owl Legends: An Archetypal Story of Creation

Table of Contents

Introduction

Stewart and Janet Swerdlow were born with their Intuition and Spiritual Connection open to their Source. They rely on their connection to bring them answers, information, and help when and where they need it, in all areas of their lives, including love, health, and finances. Through deep meditation, prayer, and much personal study, they received the symbols in this book, known as "archetypes" (pronounced *ark-a-types*).

Archetypes emanate from all things in physical reality, including your thoughts. Consciously mentally or visually using archetypes directs and amplifies their energy within your energetic field. This is like creating your own recipe rather than having the ingredients of a recipe randomly float around you.

Archetypes are geometric shapes that work in your energetic field by removing the blocks that prevent you from receiving what you truly desire and need. As these blocks come into your conscious mind, send them to your Source. Replace the blocks with the appropriate archetype to imprint and change your personal energy field, thus creating a pathway for your goals to be achieved.

Thousands of people have used these archetypes to help achieve success in all areas of their lives.

You, too, can bring what you desire and need into your life by using these archetypes to release your blocks and change your personal energy field.

The archetypes in this book are copyright protected. However, Janet and Stewart give you permission to copy these archetypes for *your personal use only* as long as you include the Expansions copyright that is included alongside each archetype, and maintain this copyright so that Expansions continues to receive credit its work.

Thank you for respecting this unique work presented to you by Janet and Stewart.

Part I

Introduction to Archetypes

1

What is an Archetype?

The Physical World is simply archetypes that appear frozen in time. Movement is archetypes in motion.

Every shape in existence is an archetype on some level. Every square, box, rectangle, circle, triangle, pyramid, and so forth is really an archetype. This is why books that teach people how to draw are full of these geometric shapes. Everything is based on archetypes, or these geometric shapes.

Dreams are filled with archetypes. When you dream, you receive these archetypes directly from your Oversoul and the Mind of God. But, since your conscious mind does not know how to interpret them, it assigns symbols that you can understand.

For example, a pink circle becomes a pink tabletop. A brown line becomes a tree. A blue oval becomes a lake. When you know how to understand archetypes, these messages that you receive from your Source become easier to interpret.

Letters of the alphabet are all archetypes/shapes. These letters/shapes represent specific sounds. The sound is a "tone," or "frequency."

Everything that exists is based upon color, tone, and archetype/

shape. For example, why is an apple an apple and not something else? Because the apple has a specific geometric shape, a specific color, and a specific tone/frequency that can only be outpictured in a specific way.

Every area of the world has food that is indigenous and unique to that place. It is easy to forget this because now, almost every food can be found somewhere. Go in any supermarket in almost any country and you will find many of the same foods.

Yet, if you go to smaller markets, you may be able to find some of the indigenous foods. Sometimes local people spend time hunting or gathering foods that are unique to their specific locale. As with all things, food is frequency.

Frequency outpictures in Physical Reality when it passes through specific geometric shapes/archetypes. This is actually very simple to understand.

Frequency is the energy stream that pours forth out of God-Mind. The flow of energy streams creates sound/tone. Just as different water flows have different sounds/tones—small creek, underground spring, raging river, raindrops—frequency flows have different sounds/tones.

The sounds/tones of the flowing frequencies generate archetypes. As the flowing frequencies pass through the archetypes, out pops the symbol of that specific energy stream into physical reality.

Nonphysical must have a gateway into the physical. This is exactly what sexuality is about—male frequency is the key that combines with female frequency to allow the nonphysical into the physical. Thus, the reason for Sexual Ritual to create in Physical Reality.

When you understand the Language of Hyperspace, which is the Original Language that emanates out of God-Mind consisting of Color, Tone, and Archetype, you, too, can consciously rearrange your archetypes to rearrange your mind-patterns. This means that you can now consciously create your world, rather than feeling like the world creates you.

2

How Do Archetypes Take Shape?

Think of pushing cookie dough through a cookie press. The raw dough is directed through a tube with a cutout shape, or archetype. When the dough is squeezed through a cookie press, out pops a cookie in the same shape as the cutout.

If you did not understand this process, looking at the finished cookie would make you wonder how the cookie arrived with that specific shape. If you looked only at the raw lump of dough beside the cookie, you might wonder how the lump of dough ever turned into a delicious, edible cookie.

The same is true of All That Exists. What kind of energetic cookie press did the frequency flow pass through to create the shapes that exist in this reality?

Archetypes are the cutouts in the cookie press that frequency flows must go through to arrive into Physical Reality.

Archetypes are the portal from the nonphysical that frequency flows must pass through to manifest into the physical.

Archetypes take their shapes from the mind-patterns of the people who exist in this reality. Why does this reality exist? Because the people who are here agree that it does.

Everyone sends out like frequency flows with their minds to create this reality.

When frequency flows are pulled out of any idea in Physical Reality, then that part of Physical Reality disintegrates, or, disappears.

For example, take any abandoned building. What caused the building to become abandoned in the first place? The people agreed that the building was no longer necessary. Once they moved out and took their mind-pattern with them, the building ceased to exist: dust to dust, ashes to ashes…it is on its way out of physical form.

Anything that is abandoned eventually disintegrates unless more thought energy is directed its way.

When you realize this process, all you have to do is mentally form an archetype-cutout, which then attracts a specific frequency flow to coalesce from the nonphysical into this Physical Reality.

3

Manifesting Nonphysical into Physical Reality

The strength of your mind-pattern determines what you can bring together for manifestation in Physical Reality.

A recipe is a recipe. Once you have the recipe, you can create. The result is not a matter of if you are "good" or "bad." The result occurs when the strength of your mind-pattern pulls your goal to you.

Here is your recipe:

- Frequency Streams Create Sounds/Tone.
- Tone Gives Frequency Streams Shapes.
- Shapes become portals from the nonphysical into the physical through which the Frequency Streams can now flow.

All Physical Reality is created via Frequency Streams emanating from God-Mind, including humans. Humans exist at the intersection of energy streams, where the physical and nonphysical meet.

The thoughts emanating from each soul-personality attracts specific Frequency Streams that create tone and form archetypes. These archetypes from the God-Mind and the archetypes from the mind-patterns meet, thus creating experience in this reality.

As a microcosm of the macrocosm, each soul-personality has Frequency Streams flowing through it, creating tone; tone shapes the frequency stream, which in turn attracts the same archetypes that flow out of God-Mind. When they match, "experience" happens.

Usually this process appears haphazard, meaning that you are not conscious of the colors, tones, and archetypes emanating from your mind-pattern. This is why chaotic thoughts create chaotic life experiences.

In addition, without appropriate boundaries the colors, tones, and archetypes of others get mixed up in your own. This results in more confusion and more chaotic life experiences that you most likely would not consciously choose.

4

Why Are Archetypes Important?

Consciously changing, directing, and re-creating archetypes changes your life experiences.

When you want to experience happiness, for example, you create new Frequency Streams within you by the words that you use. Words are spoken tone comprised of archetype. The sound is shaped depending upon the archetype used. For example the archetype "A" creates a different tone than the archetype of "B."

Each archetype allows a specific frequency to pass through it. By shaping the archetypes and sending them out, you attract the same archetype that is already floating around out there from the God-Mind.

Like attracts like. Now, you add the strength of the God-Mind to what you are already doing. This strength allows what you want to manifest. You must also utilize the wisdom of your Oversoul to determine the correctness of your desired manifestation.

By doing this, you literally re-shape the mind-pattern which then changes the archetypes that emit from you. Now, new and different archetypes from God-Mind are attracted to the emanation, resulting in new experiences due to these new archetypes.

All thought is the continued re-formulation and re-shaping of All That Is. There is never more or less to work with. All That Is remains the same. You simply rearrange All That Is by bringing the nonphysical into Physical Reality, or pass Physical Reality back into the nonphysical.

The nonphysical must be anchored into this Physical Reality. This is why you sign a contract, such as in a marriage. You have a nonphysical idea of joining two lives together. The contract provides the physical anchoring.

This is also why the indigenous peoples always make a physical offering when they take something from the physical world. They release something from the physical into the nonphysical to maintain balance. The offering signifies their honoring and acknowledgment of this process.

If you take something from the physical then you must give something back. The Mind of God is always in balance. With knowledge, you control the balance in life; without knowledge, life controls the balancing of you.

5

You Already See Archetypes

Everyone already sees archetypes. But, people have been de-focused away from this realization via "selective sight." You know what "selective hearing" is. When you are in a crowded room selective hearing allows you to tune out the background sounds to focus on one conversation.

"Selective sight" works the same way. For example, a baby's eyes look all around a person's head. Parents teach the child to focus on a nose, mouth, eyes. The child's selective sight takes over, pushing aside the archetypes to say the words that please the parents. So, from one generation to the next, selective sight is installed as the norm. No one does this "to" you. You, and generations before you, do it to your Self and to your children.

Eventually the child's eyes are trained to look right through the archetypes into the more dense areas of physical manifestations, such as the body. Some maintain archetype knowledge and sight, but few survive this selective sight process. If they do see things that the parents cannot see, then the child is off for tests and medication.

Archetypes in ancient times, when life forms were less physical, were not only more used and understood, but they were integrated and respected as a living, breathing part of life. If you were frightened of heights, an energetic archetype of courage was placed on a corresponding body part. The archetype re-directed the energy flow to negate the fear archetype, directing the energy flow to a mind-pattern of fearlessness or courage. The archetype stayed until its energy was used up; then it disappeared.

Indigenous peoples still to this day decorate their bodies and surroundings according to what they need to do. These rituals are carried forward from generation to generation. In a way, when you celebrate your own holidays and traditions, you are re-creating remnants of ancient rituals that actually meant something via color, tone and archetype.

These types of dynamic archetypes were the forerunners of today's tattoos and other body piercings and markings. The difference is that the body markings and piercings were dynamic. Today, they are static—meaning that once they are there, they are permanent. And, the inks and ink carriers are often full of chemicals and metals that are toxic to the human body.

Even if piercings are allowed to close, the energy stream is permanently disrupted unless the mind-pattern directs healing of the scarring. Sometimes it can enhance an energy flow, like an earring on the earlobe for the eye meridian to help you see better, but again, you must know what you are doing and why. This rarely happens haphazardly.

This is the same with surgeries and other more life-saving procedures. Tattoos and piercings do not allow the original mind-pattern to function, unless they represent a mind-pattern already within your psyche.

Archetypes have always been important. That is why businesses always have a logo. It is an archetype statement of what the business is that imprints your subconscious mind. For example, Target stores are a global chain of small department stores with the logo of a bright red circle with a bright red dot in the middle. The archetype of royal blue circle with a royal blue dot in the middle is the pineal gland, which represents your center of consciousness.

So, why does Target use the archetype for the pineal gland/center of consciousness for their logo, except in bright red?

Bright red is a sexual color and is found at the root chakra. Every time you look at the Target logo, you are imprinting your subconscious mind that shopping at Target will bring you sexual gratification. Target has nothing to do with sexual gratification—it is not a house of prostitution. But, by choosing this logo, your subconscious reacts and responds.

This is only one example of many. But first, you must understand your own archetypes so that you can understand the world around you.

6

Archetypes are Multidimensional

When you see an archetype on paper or on a sign, you see a two-dimensional representation of something that is in True Reality, multidimensional.

You can mentally envision the two-dimensional representation of any archetype at your pineal gland to activate it within your mind-pattern.

With eyes closed, observe the archetype. It may change color, position, and even shape. It may rotate or move around. Observe how you feel.

Ask your Oversoul to direct you as the archetype changes.

Ask your Oversoul:

- Is this a positive or negative action?
- What does this mean about my current mind-pattern?
- Does this enhance or negate my goal?
- How does this make me feel?

If you are not sure, use this affirmation:

My Oversoul now directs my understanding of this archetype, or it is removed.

Everything in existence is multidimensional. Your body is multidimensional. Each cell sends messages to your brain about what is going on within it every nanosecond. Nothing works in a straight line. Everything comes at you from a variety of directions.

You are taught linear logic during your educational process. Therefore, you expect a multidimensional life to have linear consequences. This simply does not happen.

This explains why some circumstances suddenly seem to appear from nowhere and you do not know how it happened. Again, this is because you are trying to explain a multidimensional world with linear logic.

God-Mind is not linear. God-Mind is extremely multidimensional and beyond. This is the time to remember where you came from; to acknowledge your multidimensional existence and to learn "multidimensional logic."

You are a microcosm of the macrocosm. You are a wave upon the ocean. It is time to erase the illusion that you can ever be disconnected from your Source.

As a microcosm of the macrocosm, it is time to emulate the thinking process of your Source to understand your Source rather than fall into the trap of human-designed linear logic.

As you move into multidimensional thinking, you move back into the Original Language that emanates from the Mind of God: Color, Tone, Archetype/Symbol.

More importantly, you understand the Language of your Origin.

How empowering is this?

You already work with Color, Tone, and Archetypes/Symbols, but you do it on a subconscious level. You create with them every day.

Now, with conscious awareness, you are going to create your own

Personal Recipe in a way that enhances and uplifts you into your next level of Being.

Be prepared—because the old must break up and fall away to clear the ground for a new foundation.

This is part of the process. Keep Self in alignment with Oversoul and God-Mind, and all will be well in your world. You may not always get what you want, but you will always get what you need.

The next step is to align need with wants with the wishes of your Oversoul and God-Mind.

This Trinity of Self, Oversoul, and God-Mind is the Triangle of Perfect Manifestation in Physical Reality.

You are More Than You Realize.

There is no time to lose.

Now is the Time to know who and what you are, as well as where you came from and where you are going.

Appreciate the process, for you will never pass this way again in the same way, with the same people with the same inner and/or outer circumstances.

Working with archetypes allows you to be the Powerful Co-Creator of your Destiny that you came here to be.

Prepare for change as you move your Conscious Mind into the Wonderful World of Archetypes.

7

How to Use Archetypes

Archetypes enhance your level of well-being in every area of your life.

Use them as energetic shovels to dig out what you no longer need so you can find what is causing your discomfort, observe it, learn from it, and pass it back to your Source.

Then, you must replace what you no longer need with something you *do* need. Removing anything leaves empty space. If you do not fill in the empty space with something positive, the negative will simply keep coming back.

Sometimes, there is a part of you that is afraid to let it go because that part of you prefers the what it knows to what it does not know.

Even positive change can be scary. If you have never tasted a red apple, a green apple might seem sweet. So a part of you does not want to give up the green apple.

When you realize this, it is important to remember to persevere. If you are going into places within that you have not consciously visited before, there are parts of your Self that may feel threatened and intimidated.

That is okay. There is no judgment, only observation. Continue to do your work, knowing that you are doing the best that you can with the experience you have. This life is not about being perfect. It about understanding and exploring the process.

These archetypes help you in your Self-exploration. They are not "cure-alls," but rather they are a boost to your mind-pattern.

Allow the energy of the archetypes to permeate your mind-pattern, energy field, cellular structure and surroundings.

You can visualize them at the pineal gland and then give them up to your Source, allowing them to energetically expand and or replicate as needed. These archetypes then emanate their specific frequencies out into your energy field and environments to help change your mind-pattern and thus, your life.

You can also draw them, or use Expansions' ready-made small or large templates as a visual aid to enhance your mental work. These archetypes focus specific nonphysical frequencies into the physical to enhance your ability to manifest positive changes and improvements in all circumstances. Many people report that they immediately feel the frequencies around them change to their benefit simply by having this book!

You can place the templates around your home, under your pillow, pocket, purse and/or wallet. You can put them under your water glass or bottle to absorb the frequency that you then can drink.

You can even experiment with stacking them to create powerful archetype sentences.

For example, place the Expansion Archetype on top of the Happiness Archetype. This creates an archetype sentence that says:

I expand my Happiness.

You can stack the Power Archetype on top of the New Beginnings Archetype and then add the Overall Healing Archetype. This creates an archetype sentence that says:

I now have Powerful New Beginnings that bring Overall Healing.

You can easily create your own archetype sentences or use the ones at the ones in the "Simple Archetype Sentences" section of the book to enhance and boost your mind-patterns changes.

Whatever you do, enjoy the process into Self. Always remember, as stated in *Decoding Your Life*—

YOU are the most fascinating person that you know!

Part II

Archetypes

Bear Frequency

Increases protective nature; enhances introversion for self-study; best for males however women can use this.

Affirmations

I go into the cave of my mind for Self-Study.
I now access information within to bring out to the physical world.

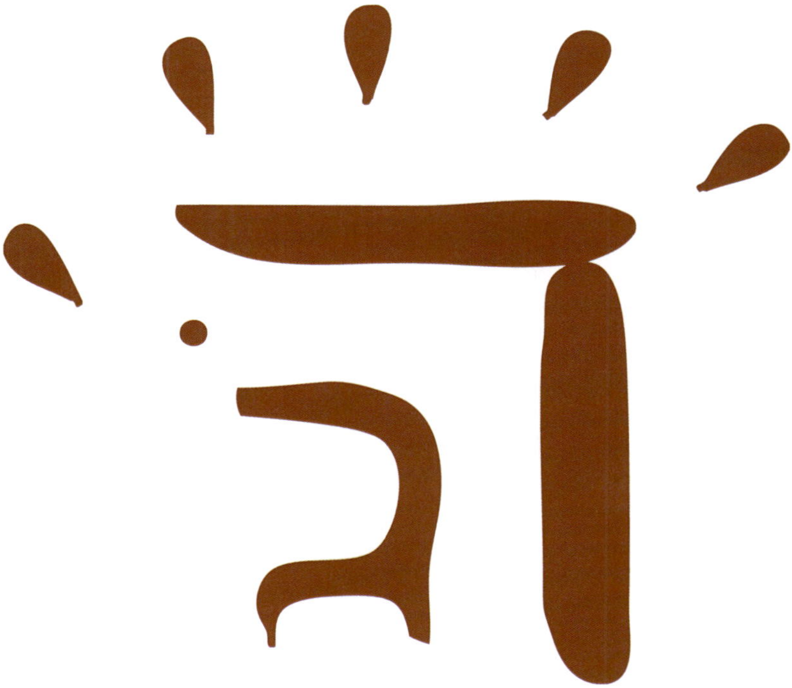

This energy is recommended more for males than females because of the body changes that usually accompany this frequency. Over time, the body becomes hairier and thicker, hands and feet enlarge, and appetite becomes ravenous, often craving dense protein.

Male genitalia enlarge and the voice deepens. There may even be an increase in height. The body may prefer extreme cold and want lots of privacy, replicating the frequencies need to go into a cave. The bear energy that you access makes the individual more protective of his partner, often increasing jealousy.

Sex becomes incredible due to its intensity. The Bear Frequency causes extremely deep penetration and long staying power. Both partners need to rest afterward, so only use the Bear Frequency when you have time to sleep and refresh yourself. One side effect is that there is a psychological need for many partners.

This obviously does not work in a committed relationship, so use this frequency sparingly if you are married or engaged. On a mental level, the Bear Frequency helps the user reach deep within the mind to retrieve information needed for use in the physical world. This causes deep reflection and contemplation so that correct decisions are made in a timely fashion.

Heavy use can also cause the personality to be argumentative. Going deep within the mind to find your solutions makes you feel right all of the time. This is a good frequency for law enforcement and military personnel, as well as politicians.

Breasts

Enhances healthy breasts for Men and Women; increases nurturing qualities.

AFFIRMATIONS

I easily nurture Self.
I accept and deserve my own Self-nurturing.

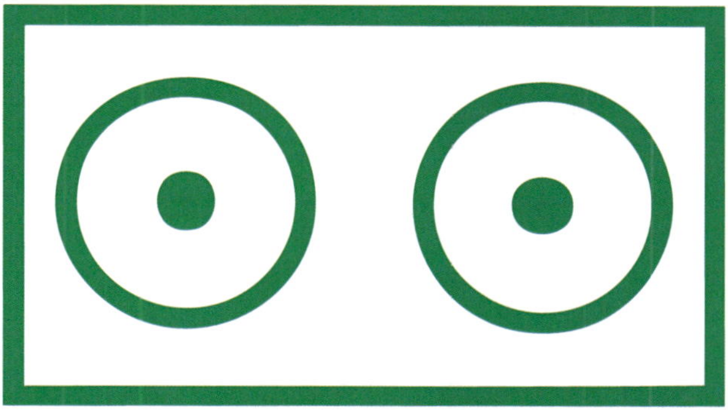

Mentally place the Breasts Archetype at the pineal to focus on Self-nurturing. Many people give to others, but forget to give to Self.

To enhance chest/breast health, mentally place the Breasts Archetype into the Medium Green Chakra Band in the chest area.

Cancellation

Removes anything unwanted from physical or nonphysical existences; always use in lower chakra colors because this is a Cancellation Archetype. Brown is the most effective color.

AFFIRMATIONS

I now "brown X" out all unnecessary negativity from my life.
I now "brown X" out *(fill in the blank),* ***according to the wishes of my Oversoul and God-Mind.***

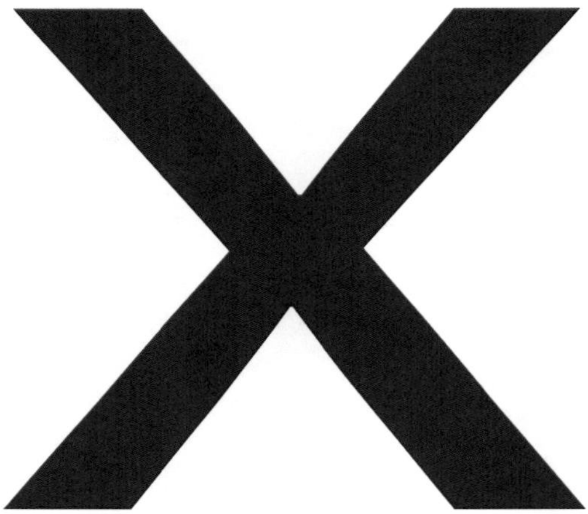

Mentally place a brown X over anything that you do not want in your life, allowing your Oversoul and God-Mind to make the final decision. If the person, place or thing disappears from your life, then this is what is most correct and beneficial for you.

If the person, place or thing remains in your life, then you still have more lessons to learn. Only move on when the lessons are learned, otherwise the lessons only become more challenging.

Communication

Speaking up as appropriate, tactfully and honestly; promotes effective communication in relationships, work, environment; standing up for your Self; voicing your opinion in a way that others can hear; speaking what is on your mind; aids public presentations; may be used to communicate with the departed or nonphysical entities as well as animals and insects with the correct animal/insect archetypes.

AFFIRMATIONS

I now easily and effectively communicate my thoughts and opinions.

I now easily and effectively communicate with *(fill in the blank).*

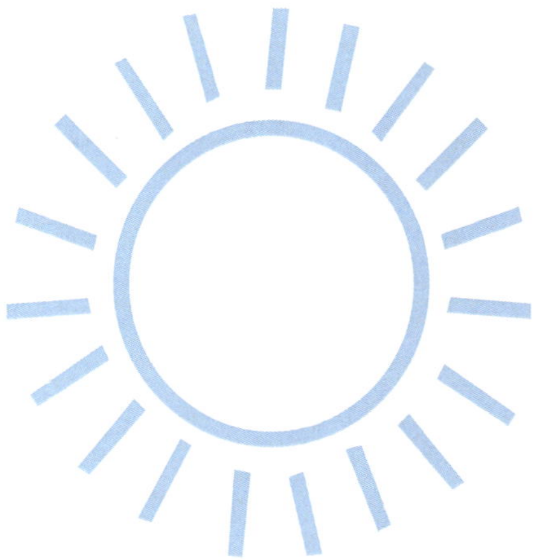

Visualize a mental picture of this Communication Archetype at the throat area. Hold the Communication Archetype at the throat area whenever you feel the need to enhance your vocal communications.

Dolphin Frequency

Eases mental shifting into Hyperspace; can be used as a sleeping aid when combined with breathing exercises at night; aids communication with and for autistic people; aids mental communication with dolphins; enhances a strong mental and physical connection between sexual partners

Affirmations

I easily move into Dolphin Frequency to aid my mental processes.

Dolphin Frequency spiritually bonds me to my partner on all levels.

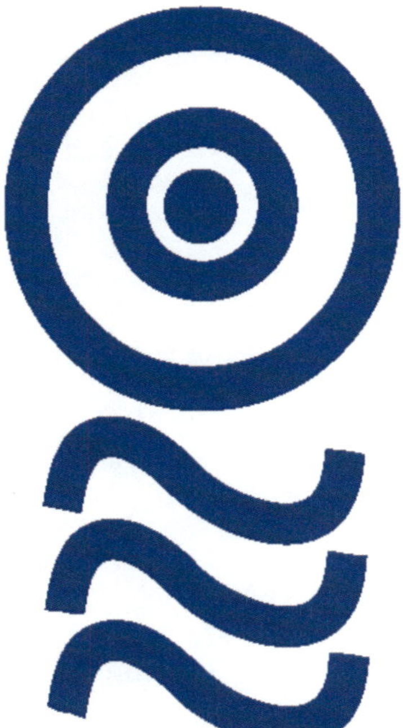

The Dolphin Frequency is unique because it is not an animal species-mind per se. The brain capacity of a dolphin is actually larger than that of a human. This means that dolphins are more intelligent than humans and also higher up on the evolutionary scale.

As with the energies of all species, dolphin energy exists on many different levels simultaneously. This means that there are both physical and nonphysical aspects to the frequency.

Holding the Dolphin Frequency Archetype at the pineal gland in royal blue during the sex act causes an automatic shifting of the energies to a hyperspace level in such a way that you feel totally like a nonphysical energy and completely protected.

This enhances the thought-form as it is projected at the moment of orgasm.

Physically, more body fluids are produced. The body feels more streamlined and easily moves through sexual positions. Using this frequency increases the likelihood of pregnancy. With this frequency, the time of the sexual act is shortened, while the spiritual feelings last for a very long time.

The Dolphin Frequency enhances a strong mental and emotional connection between the partners to such a degree that they can even know what the other thinks and feels. A closer family bond is created, as well as a deep sense of peace and understanding.

Autism is a result of active Dolphin Frequency and Dolphin DNA in that person. Use the Dolphin Frequency to communicate with autistic people and do healing work on them. Autistic people usually respond well to the Dolphin Frequency Archetype.

Emotional Balance/Pineal Gland

Actual natural archetype for the Pineal Gland; balances both hemispheres of the brain; balances endocrine/hormonal systems; aids in the correction of physical, mental, emotional, spiritual imbalances, including weight.

Affirmations

My body, mind, and emotions are now in balance.

My outer life reflects my inner balance.

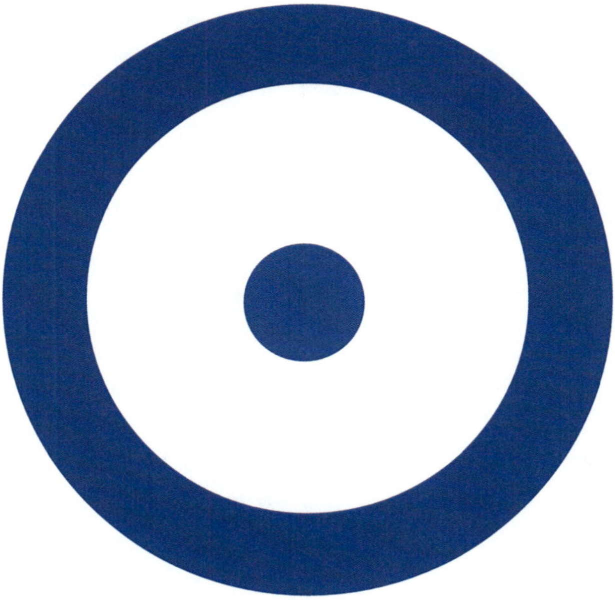

Visualizing this Pineal Gland Archetype at the pineal gland maintains brain balance. Use this whenever you feel overly emotional or too mental. Check throughout the day, and even night if you are awake, to make sure that the archetype is in place.

Expansion

Increases and expands goals and desires; use in higher Chakra colors; violet is the best; great for Radionics to increase template power; enhance mind-patterns or anything that you want.

Affirmations

My positive life experiences now expand.

I expand my abilities to fulfil my role and function in this lifeline.

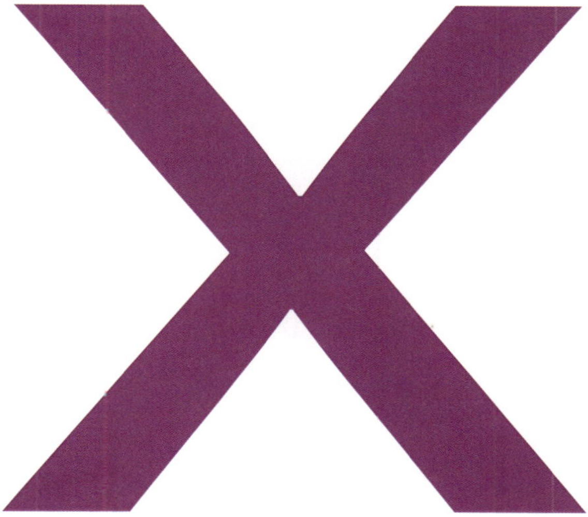

Visualize the Expansion Archetype to expand and enhance any positive circumstance from your health to wealth and from relationships to careers. This archetype is a fabulous booster for all areas of your life, both physical and nonphysical.

Female Orgasm

Removes female frigidity; increase sexual responsiveness; can help increase the potential for pregnancy.

AFFIRMATIONS

I am now sexually warm and responsive.

I am open to new ideas and new life.

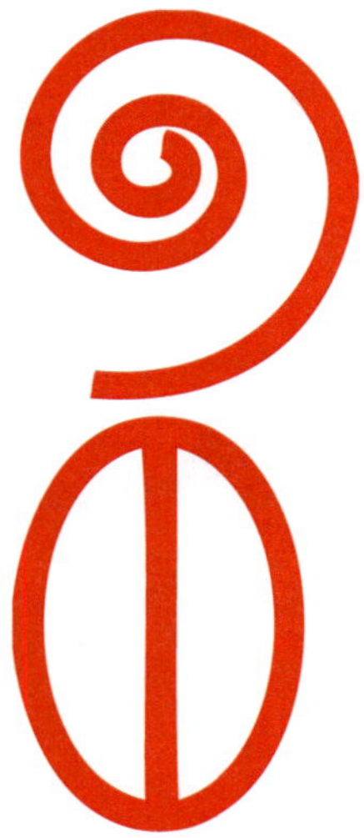

Visualize the Female Orgasm Archetype at the pineal gland as well as in and through the sexual area. With verbal or Oversoul permission, one partner can place these archetypes on/in the other partner to enhance its effectiveness.

God-Mind

All That Is; the grandparent of your Soul; your Original Source; use to guide every aspect of your life along with your Oversoul.

Affirmations

I let go and I let God.

I allow my Source to guide me at all times.

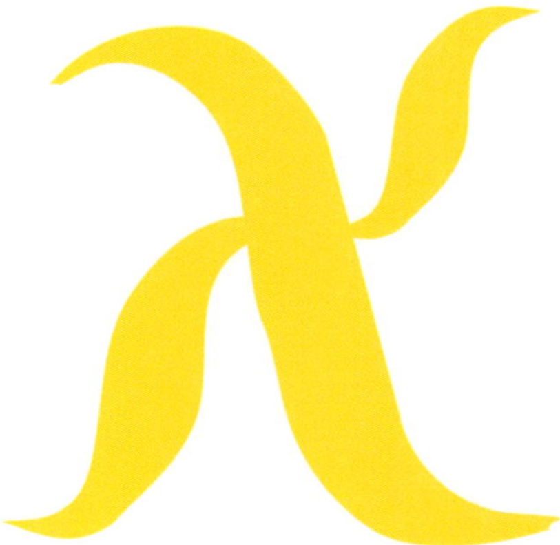

Whenever you use the Oversoul Archetype, place the God-Mind Archetype above that to form the trinity of Self, Oversoul and God-Mind. When you align with your Source, you will be exactly where you are supposed to be at all times.

Always keep Self anchored deeply within your Oversoul and God-Mind to stay centered, calm and balanced. Acknowledge your Source to acknowledge strength of Self, knowing that like a tree, you bend in the wind, but you never break. You are flexible and know how to flow with whatever Source brings to you at all times.

Happiness

Promotes feelings of Well-Being; use for love, family, friends, work, home, weight, health, body, talents, hobbies, sports, finances.

Affirmations

I am One with Happiness.

Happiness floods my Soul.

With a few adjustments in your thinking process, you can easily bring happiness and satisfaction to all areas of your life. Too often, people think that their happiness depends on what the outer world gives them.

By gently fine-tuning that thought, you realize that your happiness depends on what you project out into the world. You can use the strength of your thoughts to pull to you exactly what you need to create Happiness and satisfaction in your life.

Sometimes what you think will bring you happiness, does not, so you go from one thing to the next, looking, looking, looking. For this reason, it is important that you use the Happiness Archetype to help re-arrange your thoughts.

If you think a particular person will make you happy, mentally place the Happiness Archetype over that person's name or face every time you think of him/her. If this is not the correct person for you, the name or face will fade from your vision as it starts re-arranging your thoughts for a better person to enter your life.

Use this same process with any area of your life into which you would like to bring happiness. Combine this visualization with one or both of the affirmations, and watch your life change for the better.

What you want may need some revisions on a deeper level than you can consciously envision. The Happiness Archetype helps you determine what you really want, as well as helps bring it to you.

Individualized Consciousness

Helps you surpass the group/species mind and animal mind; recognizing your own Spark of Divinity within the God-Mind; helps you move into and stay in your Higher Mind; aids release of addictions.

Affirmations

I AM Individualized Consciousness.

I AM a unique cell of Individualized Consciousness within the God-Mind.

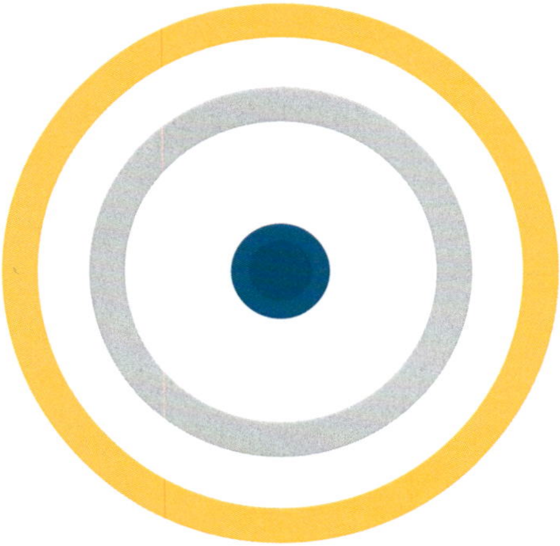

Hold this archetype at the pineal gland when you feel pressured to be a part of any group to which you do not want to belong. This archetype also helps pull out of your animal mind and into your Higher Mind.

Using this archetype also helps move you through any addictive behavior from physical addictions such as alcohol, drugs, pornography, and sex to mental/emotional addictions such as drama, argumentativeness, victim-mentality.

Leadership

Attain Self-Leadership; aids dependence on Self, Oversoul, God-Mind/Source; increases Self-confidence; enhances Self-inspiration; develops interdependence; aids your ability to "know by knowing."

AFFIRMATIONS

I AM the Leader of my Self.

I lead my Self deeper into my Source.

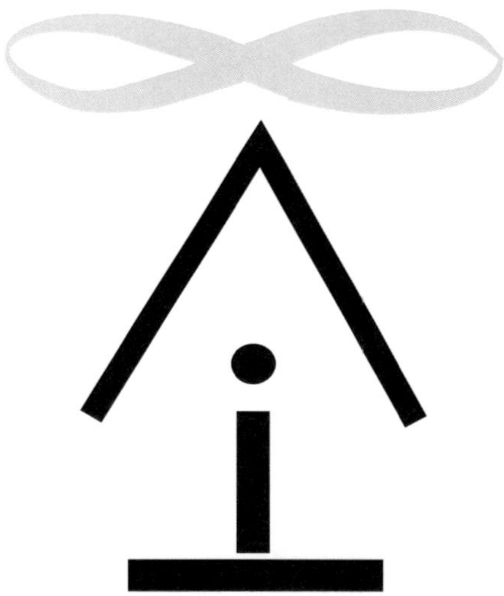

Place this at the pineal gland whenever to boost your Self-confidence in any situation. Know that you are already a leader within the God-Mind. This archetype enhances your own inner abilities to know your own strengths and weaknesses without judgment or criticism so you can enhance your weaknesses, balance your strengths and when appropriate, surround your Self with others who create an effective team.

Lion Frequency

Increases your direct awareness to God-Mind power; the highest frequency that still connects between physical and nonphysical; empowerment; protection; strength.

Affirmations

The Lion Frequency rises within me, empowering and strengthening me on all levels.

The Lion Frequency permeates my environment, powerfully protecting my inner and outer space.

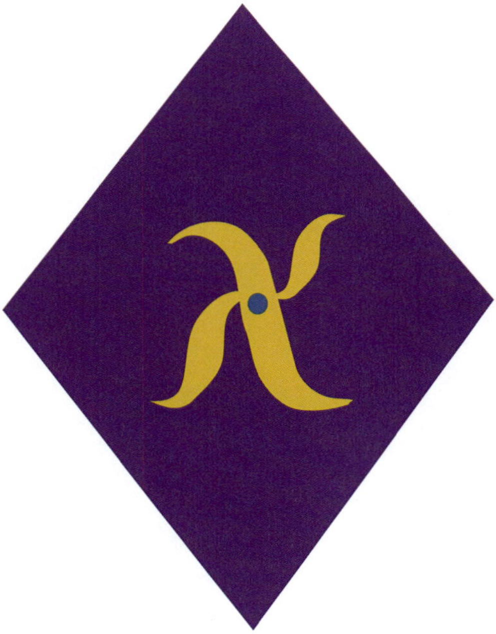

The Lion Frequency is the highest frequency that can possibly fit into physical reality. In its purest form, which takes on the appearance of a golden winged lion, there is a direct awareness of God-Mind and power. This frequency, unlike all of the others, is used at the crown chakra since it fits at the highest point of the body. The Lion Frequency gives the soul-personality a feeling of power, strength, all-knowingness, wisdom, and the ability to blend into All That Is.

Physically, using the frequency enlarges the genitalia and allows for multiple, powerful orgasms. The body becomes hairier with larger shoulders and shoulder blades, with a narrower waist. You move faster, crave proteins, and prefer cool shade, although like warm weather.

Males start comparing their bodies and strength to other men. Both male and females feel a greater affinity with nature and an even greater affinity with cats, desiring to have a lot of space around them. You may feel the sensation of wings on your shoulder blades and may find that you do not speak much, but when you do, itis powerful and meaningful. Orgasms will almost force you to roar!

The female on this frequency wants to be with like-minded females, while the male prefers to be alone most of the time. The male and female both become very fertile but the male will not really want to participate in rearing the children. Both want frequent sex, and at the moment of orgasm may have the desire to roar. Whatever is projected out while on this frequency will be amazingly enhanced and perfect. You will amaze yourself!

Logos Christos

Healing generator on specific body locations; can be used in the color of each chakra when placed there; enhances alternative healing techniques.

Affirmations

Every part of my body is now healed at all times.

My energies are balanced and radiating out for healing.

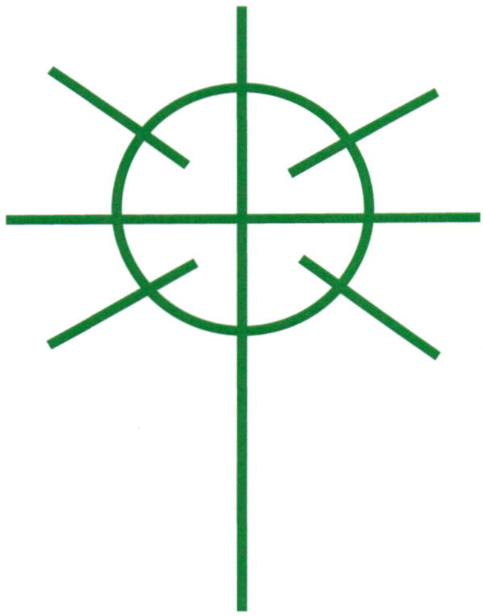

This powerful healing archetype specifically enhances all healing, both physical and nonphysical. Place it in the chakra band where healing needs to occur in the color of that specific chakra band. If you have a specific organ, body part, or system that needs healing, mentally visualize it in that location. Allow the archetype to permeate whatever needs healing.

Male Orgasm

Removes impotence; increases virility; increases fertility; enhances pregnancy possibilities; increases sperm count.

Affirmations

I now recreate the powers of the God-Mind to manifest in my Reality.

I now have an abundance of sperm to successfully bring a child into fruition.

Male Fertility

Hold mental picture of this archetype in the scrotum area. With permission, both you and your partner can mentally hold it here during sexual activity to increase virility.

Mental Balance

Creates mental balance in all mind-patterns and emotions; use in the colors of the chakra bands for balancing energies of those locations; aids deactivation of programming triggers and in deprogramming.

Affirmations

My thoughts and emotions are perfectly balanced at all times.

My mind is now in perfect balance.

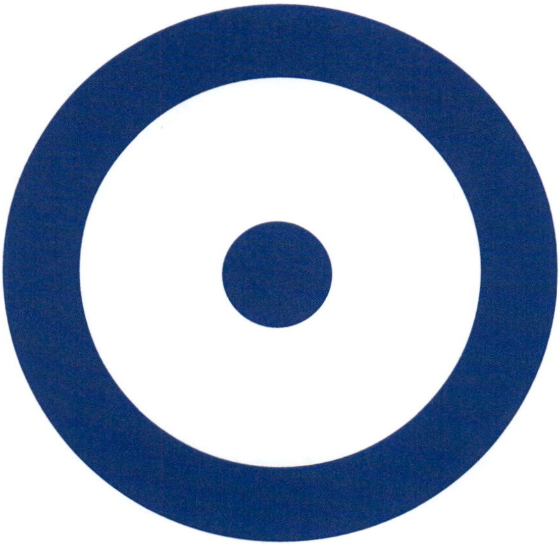

Whenever you feel like your thinking process is out of balance or your emotions are taking over, place this archetype at the pineal gland to bring your mind back to a point of balance. Focusing on this archetype helps close down programming triggers, bringing you back to reality. Balancing the brain aids in the healing of anything perceived as a mental illness.

Maltese/Magdalene Cross

Original Symbol of Creation; represents the four elements of the Earth coming together at a central location; use to access and open genetic memory for this time period.

AFFIRMATIONS

I now access my genetic memory from this time period if it is correct and beneficial.

I now understand my Simultaneous Existences from this time period in a way that is most correct and beneficial.

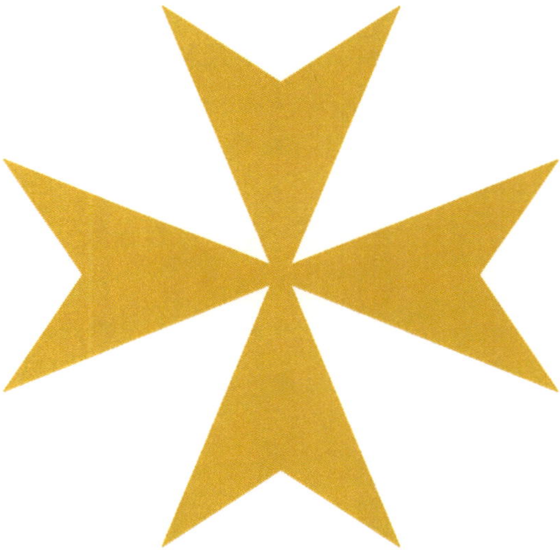

Use this archetype to access and open genetic memory from this time period. If you do not receive any information, then it is not correct for you to know at this time, or, you do not have lifelines in this time period. Refer to Maltese/Magdalene Cross Visualization in *Hyperspace Plus*.

Merging with Aspects of Alternative Selves

Use to pull into this Physical Reality traits and characteristics that are desirable from your alternate realities. Bring current goals to fruition by merging with your Self in the Eternal Now.

AFFIRMATIONS

I now merge with all my alternate selves in every universe where I exist where (fill in the blank with what you want to bring in or enhance)

I now merge with all my alternate selves in every universe where I exist with whatever is most correct and beneficial for all involved with the guidance of my Oversoul and God-Mind.

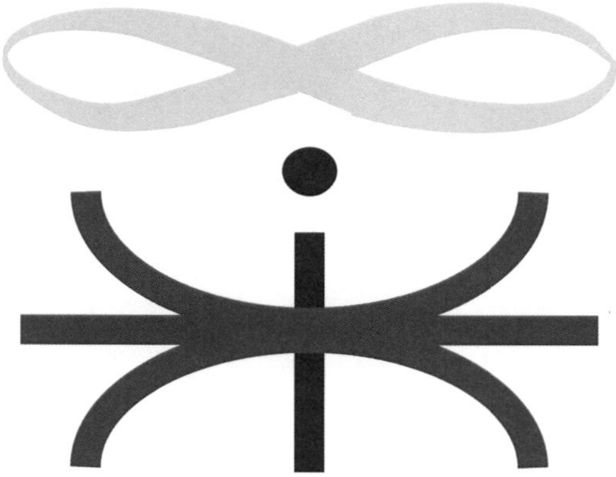

Place this archetype at your pineal while visualizing whatever it is that you want to pull in from other realities. *Hyperspace Plus* has a detailed visualization if you would like to explore the use of this archetype on a deeper level.

New Beginnings

Start new projects as well as helps make old/current situations like new, such as relationships, health, finances, residence, career, talents, hobbies, children, school, relocation, prosperity.

AFFIRMATIONS

I successfully initiate New Beginnings in all appropriate areas of my life.

I have successful New Beginnings in (fill in the blank.)

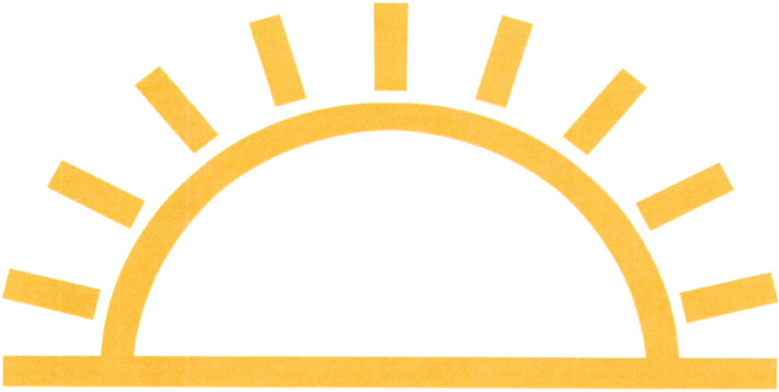

How many times in your life have you tried to implement New Beginnings? If you are finally ready to accept positive successful New Beginnings in your life, it is important that you follow these simple recommendations:

- Make a list of all the areas in which you would like New Beginnings.
- Focus on one area at a time.
- Achieve success in one New Beginning area.

- Feel the New Beginning imprint in your energy field increase and grow stronger.
- Be consistent in your forward movement.
- If you go backwards, release any judgment or criticism of yourself up to your Source.
- Focus on the next area until you achieve success.
- Be patient—quick fixes do not last; slow and steady win the race!

Following the above recommendations helps you successfully implement a positive New Beginning in any area of your life. With your feet on a new path, you will find another, more desirable direction that gives your life new meaning.

Overall Healing

Heals body, mind, and soul; physical mental; enhances emotional and spiritual healing in all areas of your life.

AFFIRMATIONS

I am ready for Overall Healing in my life.

I now accept and experience Overall healing throughout my entire life stream.

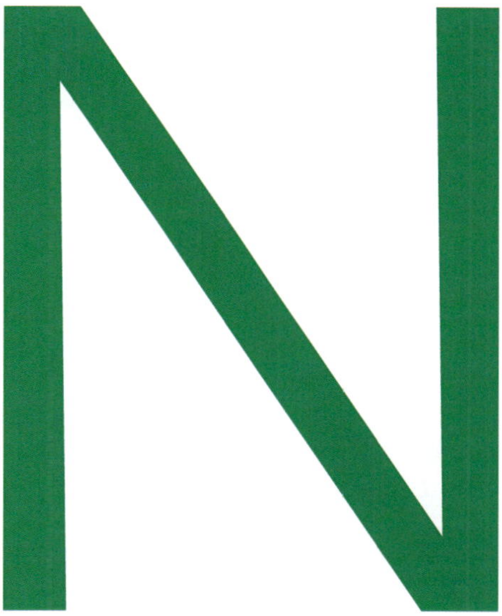

Whenever you feel like you need healing in any area of your life, visualize the Oversoul Healing Archetype throughout your entire Being and energy field. Visualize it from the ground upon which you are standing up to the top of your head. Feel it radiating and permeating every cell of your physical and nonphysical Self.

Oversoul

Your Point of Origin out of the God-Mind. The parent of your Soul; use to determine what is most correct and beneficial in thought, word and deed.

Affirmations

I align my wishes and desires with the wishes and desires of my Oversoul.

I ask my Oversoul before I open my mouth or move my body.

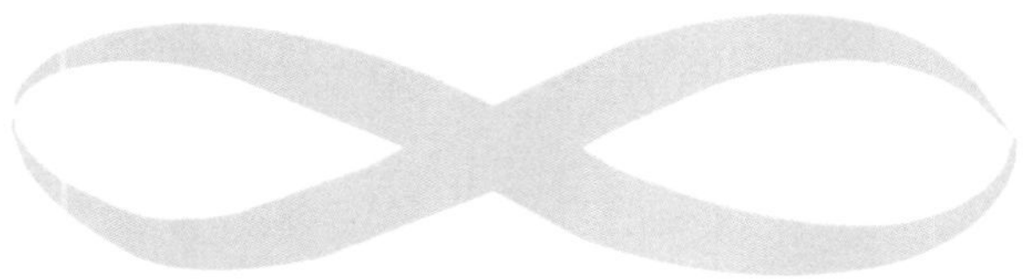

Hold the Oversoul Archetype above all of your mental work. This allows all the final decisions to be made from a higher perspective. You may not get what you want, but you will get what you need, eventually understanding why circumstances happened as they did.

Perfect Manifestation/Creation

Projection from the Mind to Create; used to ground mind-patterns into physical reality.

AFFIRMATIONS

My dreams and desires now manifest in physical reality in the way that is most correct and beneficial for me.

I give thanks for (fill in the blank), its equivalent, or something better, in accordance with the wishes of my Oversoul and God-Mind.

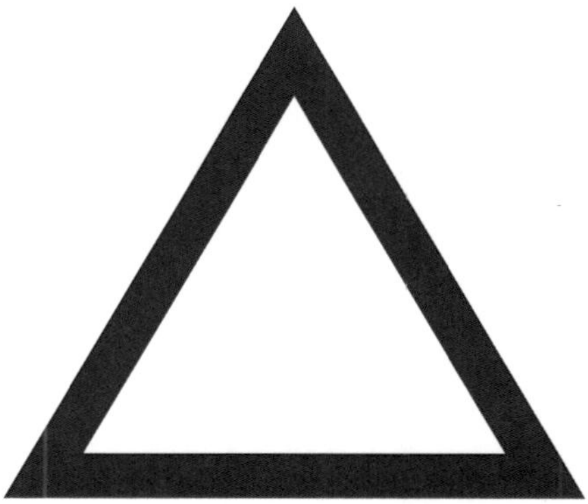

Visualize the image of whatever you desire inside the brown triangle as you say your affirmations. Remember, just because you *can* create something does not mean that it is most beneficial and correct for you. Always allow your Source to make the final decisions.

Pi, Violet

Use as the key to unlock information hidden in your DNA; can be used as a deprogramming aid.

AFFIRMATIONS

I now use the Violet Pi to unlock my DNA.

I now accurately interpret the information downloaded with the aid of the Violet Pi.

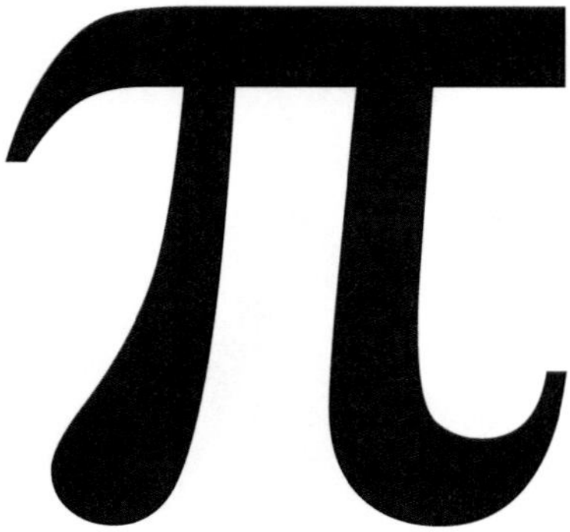

For detailed instructions, refer to the "Opening DNA with Violet Pi" visualization in *Hyperspace Plus.*

Power

Increases Personal Power in Every Aspect of Your Life; can be used in the color of a specific chakra to increase healing and/or organ function; enhance work, home, finances, relationships, health, sexuality, prosperity, relocation, talents, hobbies, sports, communication, courage.

Affirmations

I allow the Power of my Oversoul and God-Mind to flow in and through me.

The Power of my personal attributes increases in a way that I most comfortably handle.

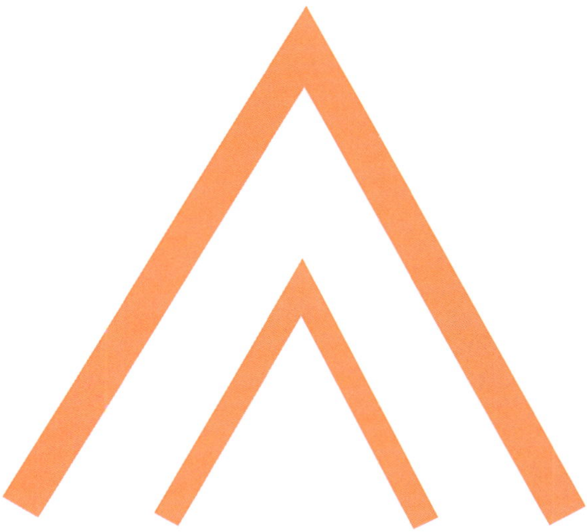

Power is your own inherent strength to bolster any physical, mental, emotional, or spiritual ability. Bring forth your Personal Power using the following visualization:

- Visualize and know that Personal Power already exists within you.
- Visualize and feel your Personal Power swell up from your depths.
- Visualize and feel your Personal Power flood every cell of your physical, mental, emotional and spiritual selves.
- Visualize and feel your Self strong and focused.
- Know that you are anchored in the midst of your own Personal Power.
- Know that anchored in this strength, you can face anything; you can accomplish anything.
- Recognize that you are in charge of all aspects of your Self.
- Tap into your Personal Power any time you desire.
- Connect with your Source to utilize your Personal Power wisely and correctly.

With focus and direction, opening up to your own Personal Power changes all aspects of your life forever. You are now responsible for your actions and reactions from a point of power. Once open, always open—your personal power is a constant flow.

Pregnancy

Increases fertility; maintain healthy pregnancy.

AFFIRMATIONS

I now achieve and maintain a healthy pregnancy.

I am now pregnant.

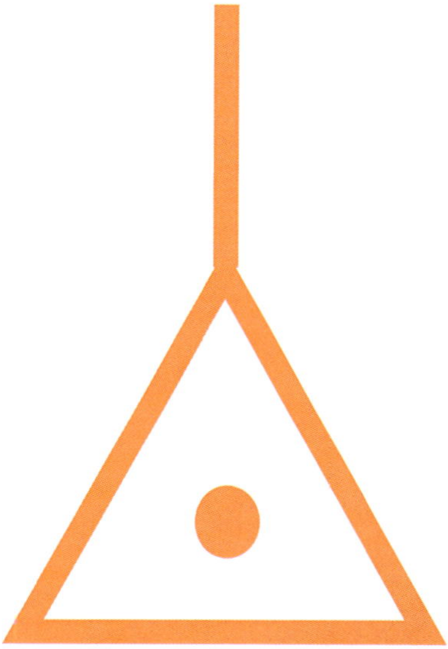

Hold mental picture of this archetype in the area of the uterus. Place template on body at the uterus. During pregnancy, continue to hold the mental picture in the uterus at all times.

Pregnancy Prevention

Prevents pregnancy without disturbing your fertility.

Affirmation

I activate the Pregnancy Prevention Archetype within my uterine area.

I mentally hold the Pregnancy Prevention Archetype within my uterus.

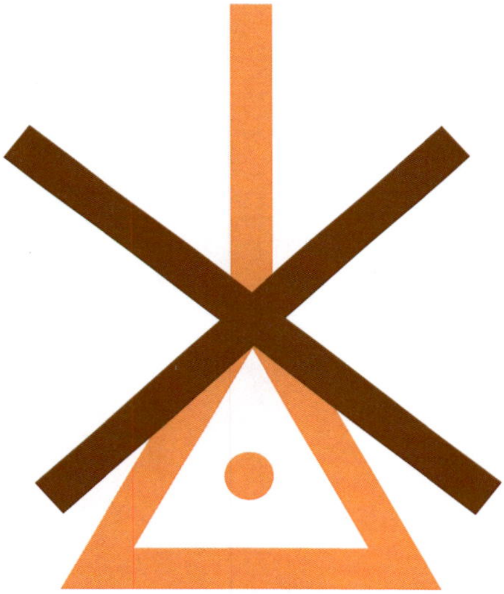

During sexual activity both partners can hold the Pregnancy Prevention Archetype in the uterine area.

Release & Resolve Past Issues

Cleans out what you no longer need; helps resolve unresolved past issues including relationships, family, career, finances, hurts, angers, bitterness, frustration, jealousies, injustices, weight, sexual abuse, abandonment, and victimization.

AFFIRMATIONS

I now resolve and release all no-longer-necessary past issues.

I now resolve and release (fill in blank with specific issue).

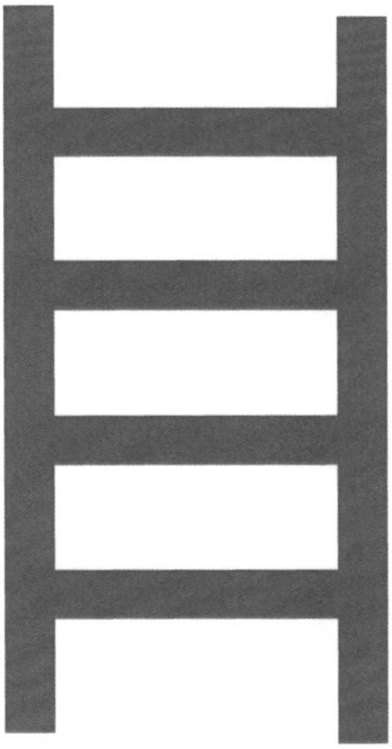

Would you finally like to get to the core of what holds you back from achieving your goals? Most likely, you have unresolved issues from your past literally weighing you down. How can you move forward when your past keeps tugging at you from behind?

You feel like one step forward and two steps back. Frustration and self-judgment/self-criticism increase while your current goal seems even further away. Time to end the cycle.

Make a list of everything from your past that bothers you. This is not about "logic," this is about "emotion" and how you feel, so do not judge what bothers you. If it bothers you, it bothers you. Put it on your list.

Mentally visualize the Release & Resolve Past Issues over each item on the list. Observe what comes forward into your conscious mind.

Pay attention to what you see, feel, or know, even if at first it feels totally unrelated to the issue.

Do not tell your Self, "I'm not getting anything," because you *are* getting something.

Ask your Oversoul to explain how what you see, feel, or know is related to your issue. You may or may not get your answer immediately.

That is okay, because you are starting the process. Sometimes it takes a while for the issues to percolate up from your depths. You may have many seemingly unrelated experiences, that when first looked at, appear unrelated.

This can be like looking at a tree. if you look at the branches on one side of the tree you may not realize that there are branches on the other side. You have to step back to realize that there are many branches, all on the same tree trunk.

This is usually the way it is with issues. Usually, on the deeper levels, they have the same tree trunk and buried roots. This is why it is important to never say "I'm not getting anything."

Keep looking and asking questions. There is a reason for whatever you get, no matter how small or unrelated it appears at the time.

Make your notes and eventually the larger picture will come into focus so that you can finally clear the origin of your issue and move on.

Use these affirmations to help propel you forward.

Draw and carry your Release & Resolve Past Issues Archetype with you, or use one of "Expansions'" archetype cards. Sleep with it under your pillow and/or put it under your water glass to absorb the frequency. This helps to rearrange your mind-pattern so you *can* let go of what you no longer need, creating space for what you currently need, allowing positive, progressive changes to manifest into your life.

Rejuvenation

For physical rejuvenation; use in conjunction with reversing the clock exercise in *Healer's Handbook*; makes physical body youthful and vibrant; promotes healing of internal organs.

AFFIRMATIONS

My physical body reflects the agelessness of my Soul.

My physical body restructures, refines, rejuvenates and reverses the aging process.

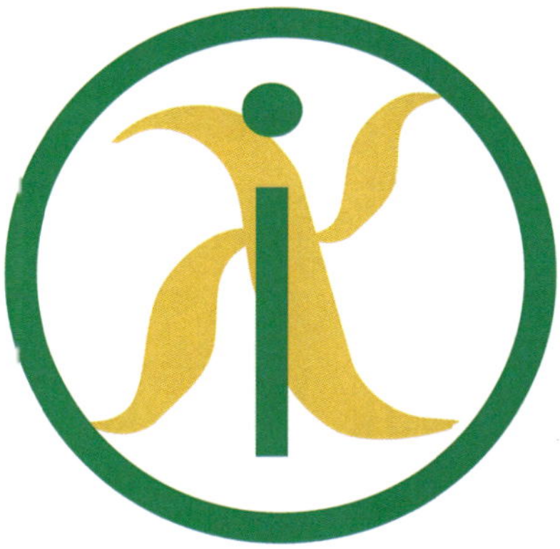

Most people believe in the "Death Program," which you can read about in Janet's Articles in *True World History.* Instead, focus on the Eternal Now, which rejuvenates your mental and emotional processes, remembering that your body follows your mind.

Visualize this archetype at the pineal gland, at any specific place within your physical body that needs rejuvenation, or visualize it mentally permeating your entire physical body from the bottom of your feet through the top of your head.

Relationships

Improves and enhances people connections; attracts the best reflection in a partner; helps heal and balance broken relationships and relationships in turmoil—personal, love, family friends, cultural, political, work, neighbors; can be used in pale pink to help repair damaged relationships.

AFFIRMATIONS

I now have healthy, positive supportive relationships.

My relationship with (fill in blank) heals and improves in a way that we both can positively handle.

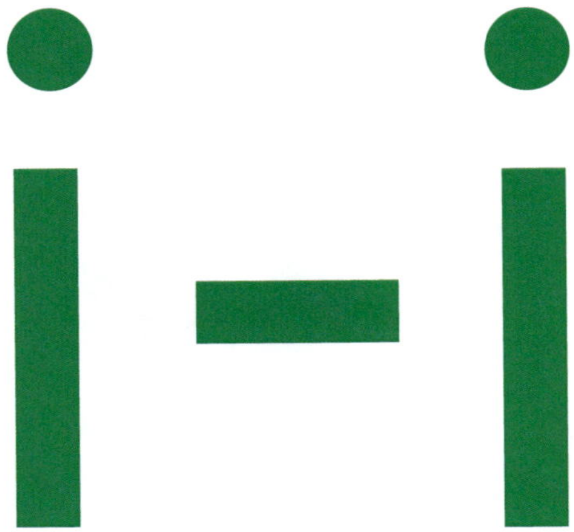

On the Oversoul level, visualize Self and the person with whom you need relationship healing. Visualize the archetype with one figure over one person and the other figure over you, with the line between you while you say the above affirmations.

Reptilian Brain Stem

Original Part of the Brain that controls the Animal Mind; balances the Reptilian Brain Stem; deprogramming; part of the White Winged Dragon Complex Archetype.

AFFIRMATIONS

My Reptilian Brain Stem is now in Balance.

I AM in control of my Animal Mind.

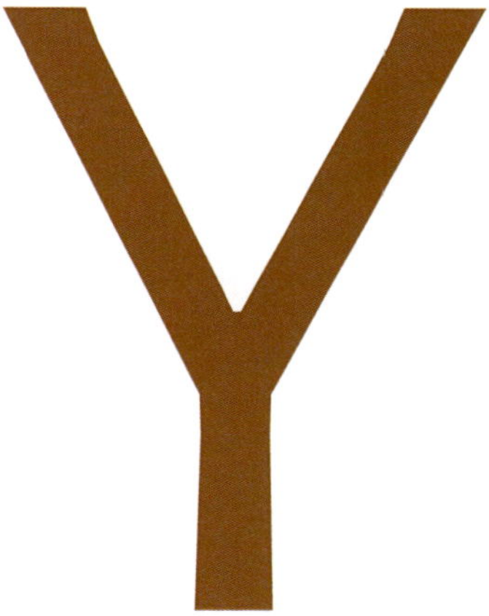

Place one part of the left arm of the "Y" in the left brain at the back of the head and the right arm of the "Y" in the right brain at the back of the head. Visualize the stem going down the back of your neck. Say your affirmations and do the appropriate mental work.

Scorpion Frequency

Deprogramming; use for deprogramming; empowering; self-defense of physical body.

Affirmations

I now powerfully control my sexual energy.

I now defend my Self fearlessly at all times.

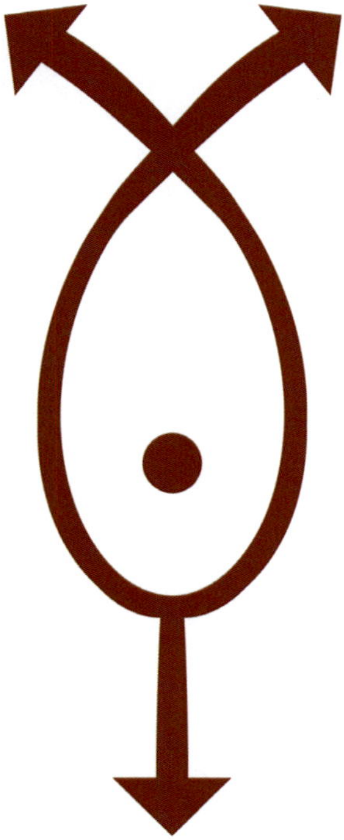

Use this archetype by placing one arrow in the left brain; one arrow in the right brain; one arrow in the coccyx bone. Next, say your affirmations and do your deprogramming work.

Self-Integration

Merges All Parts of Self into One. Use to move from Illusion into True Reality; from Compartmentalization to Oneness; Aids Deprogramming; Helps Prevent Triggering; Enhances Self-control; Mental Balance; Emotional Balance; Spiritual Balance; Focus; Obsessive-Compulsive Behavior; Decrease/ Eliminate Nightmares.

AFFIRMATIONS

I am now whole and complete in every layer of my Being.

I am One with my Source.

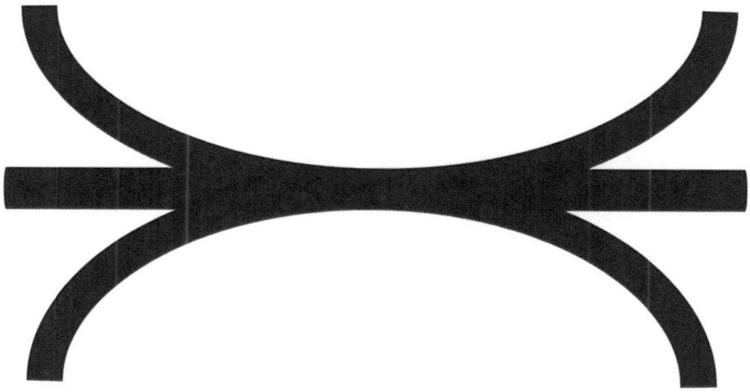

Today's world is designed to compartmentalize and divide—families, friends; cultures; even you within you; your emotions, thoughts, spiritual connections.

This perpetuates the illusion that everything is "separate" when in True Reality everything is One.

As a microcosm of the macrocosm, you can never be separate from your Source, much less from your Self. But, with the illusions in place, sometimes you may feel completely isolated from everything in existence.

Focus the Self-Integration Archetype at the pineal gland. Mentally hold it in place 24/7 so that no matter what happens in the outer world, you feel whole, complete, balanced and One with your Oversoul and God-Mind; One with All That Exists.

Throughout your day, and even your night, mentally look to make sure that this archetype stays exactly where it belongs; also that it does not float apart or turn sideways or upside down.

As long as you mentally keep the Self-Integration Archetype where it belongs you will find your life journey coming together in ways that benefit all levels of your Being.

Spiritual & Intuition Connection

Improves conscious connection with your Oversoul and God-Mind; increases spiritual connections and intuition; aids getting your own answers in all situations; helps you to be at the correct place at the correct time; helps you to meet the correct people; enhances your ability to know what to say and when to say it; improves Self-reliance and Self-confidence.

AFFIRMATIONS

I know by knowing.

I am consciously connected to my Source at all times.

Your Spiritual & Intuition Connection is one of the most important attributes that is available to you in this lifeline. When your Spiritual & Intuition Connection is open and receptive to answers from your Source, you can accomplish almost anything. At some point in your life, your Spiritual & Intuition Connection has guided you.

This can be anything from being in the correct place at the correct time, to saying the correct thing to the correct person, to just knowing what to do at the appropriate moment. This is your Spiritual & Intuition Connection doing what it does best.

You can easily and consciously open your Spiritual & Intuition Connection even further by using the correct archetype. Simply mentally place this archetype at the top of your head, and let it do the work for you. Ask a question and see what happens. Your answer always comes. Your next step is to learn to correctly interpret the answer.

Intuition may or may not have words. Your answer may be from a book that you decide to look at, a person you happen to run into, a painting on the wall, or something in Nature. When you get your answer, you simply "know." This is your Spiritual & Intuition Connection at work.

The more that you practice this technique, the more your conscious Spiritual & Intuition Connection grows. This is easy and simple, as long as you remember to do it!

Ultimate Protection

Protects person, place and thing, including you, family, friends, pets, home, car, airplane, train, bus, boat, personal property, geographic locations.

AFFIRMATIONS

I am always protected.

I am always protected wherever I go and whatever I do.

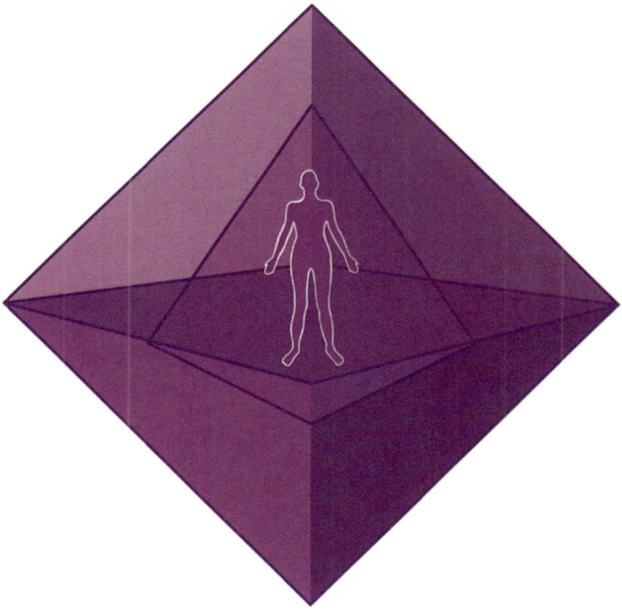

The Ultimate Protection Archetype is designed to protect whatever you place inside of it. This archetype is a geometric shape that is, according to Bible Code studies, the master shape of the God-Mind. All other shapes, archetypes, and letters can be found within it.

To most effectively use the Ultimate Protection Archetype, visualize whatever you wish to protect inside a violet tetrahedron.

Then, place this violet tetrahedron inside a violet octahedron. You may also place a gold sphere around this geometric shape.

Remember that you can mentally create the Ultimate Protection Archetype over your spouse, children, parents, relatives, boyfriend, girlfriend, friends, and even your pets! You can create the Protection Archetype over your home, homes of others, workplace, vacation location, restaurant, or where you shop.

You can also create the Protection Archetype over your modes of transportation, including car, airplane, train, bus, and boat. You can use it to help protect your personal property during storms, fires, flooding, or other natural disasters.

Use your mind to "check in" from time to time to see if the Protection Archetype is still there, or if you need to mentally re-create it again. If you see it, leave it be. If you look and it is not there, simply use your mind to re-create it again.

If you have any fears for the person, place, or thing that you would like protected, release these fears up to your Source. Immediately replace your fear thought with a picture of the Protection Archetype. Ultimately, it is up to the person, place, or thing to accept the help of the Protection Archetype. Use your mind to send out the Protection and know that it is up to the recipient to accept or reject your offerings of safety and protection.

Wealth & Prosperity

Enhances finances and life prosperity; financial wealth; increases energy; removes financial blocks; enhances creativity; increases money-making ideas; improves Self-worth; aids in increasing multiple income streams.

Affirmations

I AM now wealthy and prosperous in ways that I can most comfortably handle.

My income streams increase and multiply in ways that I can accept and incorporate into my life.

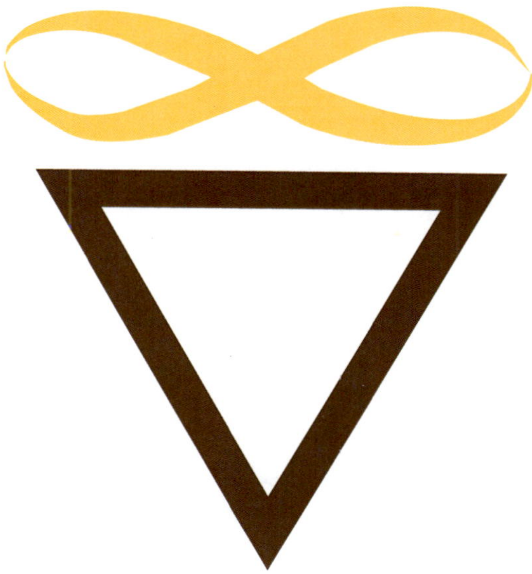

Would you like to increase your flow of Wealth & Prosperity? Would you like to be able to turn on a faucet and watch all of your desires flow into your life? Use the following visualization to increase your personal Wealth & Prosperity flow:

- Make a list of all the blocks that you perceive put limitations on your Wealth & Prosperity. Your list can include people, places, and/or things.
- Mentally visualize the Wealth & Prosperity Archetype over each perceived block.
- Hold the mental image until the block disappears and you only see the Wealth & Prosperity Archetype.
- Repeat this visualization every time you think of one of the blocks.
- One day, you will realize that the block is totally gone and no longer exists.
- Now you are able to allow Wealth & Prosperity to flow freely into your life in all areas that you desire.
- In addition, draw the Wealth & Prosperity Archetype on a piece of paper or purchase a ready-made card from Expansions. Carry the Wealth & Prosperity Archetype with you, sleep with it under your pillow, and/or put it under your water glass to absorb the frequency.

Allow Wealth & Prosperity to permeate all of your life—from your relationships to your career to your Spiritual Connection. Experience Wealth & Prosperity in every facet of your life. Turn on the faucet so you can accept the positive limitless abundance of the God-Mind. There is plenty of everything for everyone, including *you*!

Wisdom

Helps the determination of what is most correct and beneficial in all circumstances; enhances coordination of logical and creative thoughts to bring forward new improved ideas; aids the correct use of knowledge.

AFFIRMATIONS

I use my knowledge with wisdom.

Wisdom guides my thoughts, words, actions and reactions.

Hold the Wisdom Archetype at the Pineal Gland whenever you need help deciding the correct course of action for any situation. You may know what to do, but you must determine what is the most correct and beneficial course of action for all involved.

Simply because you know something does not give you the right to say what you know unless you have permission on the inner levels.

You can have a lot of knowledge, but used incorrectly it can cause a lot of damage on many levels for people, places and things.

Wisdom is the key to successfully staying on your chosen path in the way that is most correct and beneficial for you.

Wolf Frequency

Enhances family relationships; used in friendships, business associations and groups of all sorts to enhance harmony and cooperation.

Affirmations

Wolf Frequency permeates my family relationships, creating harmony and cooperation on all levels.

Wolf Frequency harmonizes my positive friendships, creating cooperation and bonding in ways that are most correct and beneficial for all.

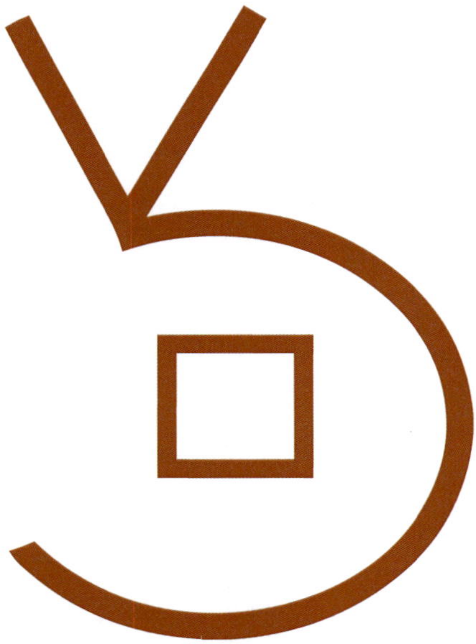

Wolf Frequency is closely associated with clan and family, enhancing the development of close family relationships, good times between people or groups of people, and camaraderie.

Wolf energy is warm and nurturing, with an aggressive side that is only excited during family crises or attacks by others. Then, the person on this frequency finds strong support and aid from those around him/her. The physical qualities of this frequency include a slim figure with lovely hair and lots of energy. The person prefers cooler weather and includes a wide mix of plants and animal proteins in his/her diet. The individual leads a more controlled and regimented life with an occasional wild time.

This frequency is generally extremely loving and caring toward others. Couples who use this sexually are devoted to one another and enjoy life together.

Wolf Frequency also helps people to understand hard times and dark energies.

Using it enables you to get yourself out of many predicaments and challenging life situations in an efficient manner. Child rearing is also made easier for those who use this frequency.

Wolf Frequency maintains a very conventional sexuality that does not go to extremes. However, the frequency is reliable, always promoting satisfaction between the couple. A sense of loyalty and respect pervades the sexual union and relationship. Wolf Frequency supports anyone who has been sexually abused or who has a fear of sex, helping him/her overcome these types of issues.

Mentally visualize the person, people, or groups at your Pinal Gland. Then, visualize the Wolf Frequency Archetype over the image to enhance harmony and cooperation. If the relationships are supposed to be, this will happen. If not, the relationships will come a part so something better can come into your life.

Part III

Nature Archetypes

Air

Helps to analyze what is in the air; to become connected to air and understand it; to understand physical breath of life; communicate with the wind; understand air movement, oxygenation, winds of change, changes of your life; aids in dream interpretation.

AFFIRMATIONS

I allow the winds of change to gently blow through my life.

The breath of life permeates my body, mind and soul.

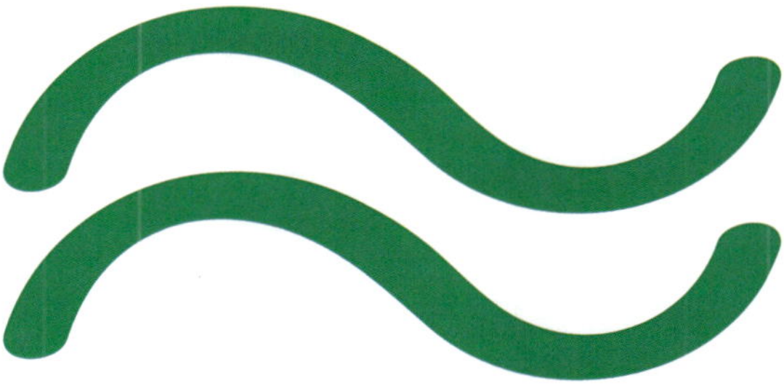

Visualize the Air Archetype at the Pineal Gland as you state your affirmations or explore your outer world. Ask the Air to explain itself to you or ask it any questions that come into your mind.

When you have dreams about anything that has to do with air, such as winds, tornadoes, hurricanes and/or storms, place the Air Archetype at the Pineal Gland to aid in your Dream Interpretation.

Earth

Feel the rhythm of the tectonic plates; volcanic activity; plant growth; minerals in the soil; grounding and balancing, aids in understanding the Mother Frequency; aids in Dream Interpretation.

Affirmations

I feel the heartbeat of the Earth.

The Mother Frequency supports and nourishes me.

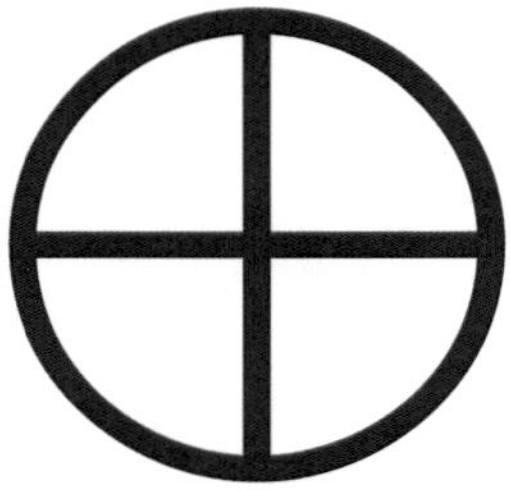

Visualize the Earth Archetype at your Pineal when you want to be connected to the Mother of your physical body. Or if you want to communicate with the Earth. The food that sustains your physical body comes from the Earth, so the Earth Archetype helps you align your physical structure with this Physical Reality. You can also use it if you want to ask the Earth questions about her history, why she exists and why humanity exists here.

The more you explore with the Earth Archetype, the more you understand this Physical Reality in its entirety as well as why you chose to be here at this time.

In addition, you can use it to help you understand any dreams that you have regarding the Earth such as earthquakes, ground upheavals, chasms, canyons, mountains, hills, and so forth. Simply place the Earth Archetype at the Pineal Gland over any dream scene that you wish to interpret and see what comes into your conscious mind.

Fire

Transmutes energy; eliminates what does not belong; reflects anger issues; can be used to create as well as destroy; purifies; aids in Dream Interpretation.

AFFIRMATIONS

I allow the Fire Frequency to show me my own internal anger issues.

The Fire Frequency purifies and transmutes my negatives into positives.

Mentally place the Fire Archetype at your pineal gland. Allow it to pull from your depths all that needs to be cleaned out or transmuted into something more positive in your life.

You can even mentally allow it to grow until it permeates and engulfs your entire being, releasing what you no longer need back to your source.

Visualize the flame turn to higher chakra colors such as:

- Pale pink to transmute negative relationships into positive ones;
- Medium green to transmute negative emotions to positive ones;
- Ice blue to transmute negative spoken and unspoken words to positive ones;
- Royal blue to transmute negative thoughts to positive ones;
- Violet to transmute harmful mind-patterns to helpful ones;
- Silver to transmute blocks to your Oversoul into stepping stones;
- Gold to transmute incorrect perceptions into wisdom.

When you have dreams about anything that has to do with fire, place the Fire Archetype at the Pineal Gland over the dream scene. See what comes up and then ask your Oversoul to interpret what this represents for you, specifically.

Lake

Use to identify specific emotional issues in life that need to be assimilated and changed/cleansed; sets and maintains emotional boundaries; aids in dream interpretation.

Affirmations

I set and maintain my emotional boundaries.

I easily identify my specific emotional issues that need to be assimilated and cleansed.

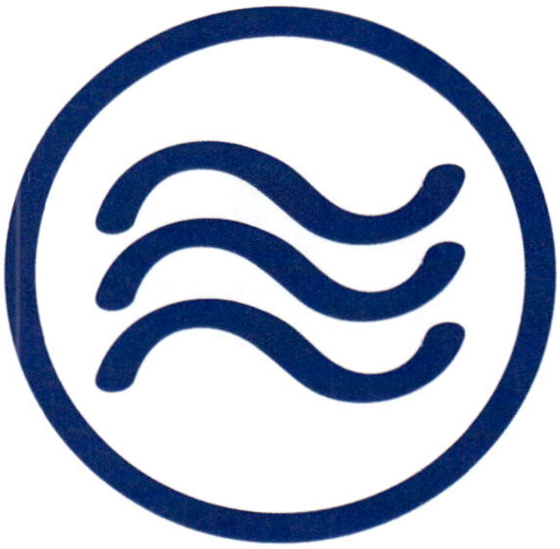

Place the Lake Archetype at the Pineal Gland to communicate with any specific lake in the outer world. The lake will communicate to you whatever you need to know about it and what it represents to you, personally.

You can also mentally visualize the Lake Archetype at the Pineal Gland and ask what emotional boundaries you need to look at and why.

And, if you have any dreams about lakes, you can place the Lake Archetype at the Pineal Gland to aid in Dream Interpretation so that you can understand the specific message that is coming to you about you, from your superconscious mind.

Sky

Use to understand the heights of your spiritual awareness and what your boundaries are in life; elevates Self to higher perspectives; connect to the atmosphere around the Earth to understand what is within and without; aids in Dream Interpretation.

Affirmations

I elevate my Self to higher perspectives and levels of Spiritual awareness.

I connect to the atmosphere of the Earth to understand my own inner atmosphere.

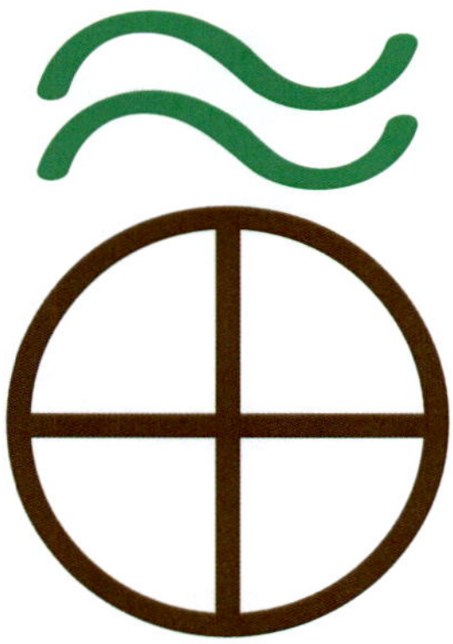

Place the Sky Archetype at your Pineal Gland as you say your affirmations. Also visualize it at your Pineal Gland when you want to connect to the Sky to find out what is in the atmosphere around the Earth and why it is there.

When you have a dream about the sky or anything in the sky that might seems strange or foreign, simply place the dream scene at your Pineal Gland and then the Sky Archetype over scene. Observe what comes up and then ask your Oversoul to help you understand what you see.

Smoke

Represents confusion in your perspective; can be used to hide things, can be used as warning signs in your life; form of communication; aids in Dream Interpretation.

Affirmations

I clearly see through my own inner smoke screens.

I clearly see through the smoke screens of others.

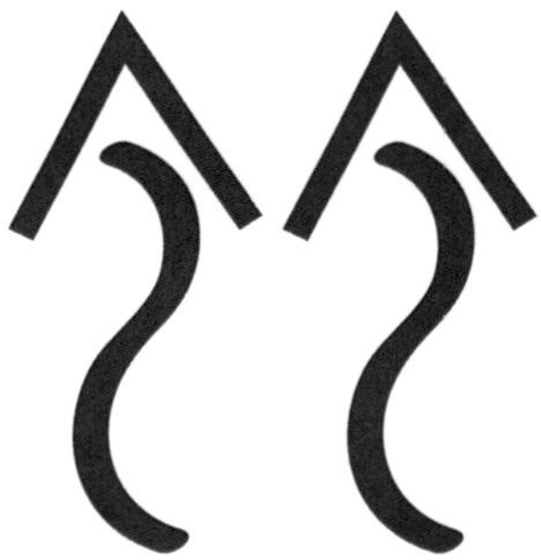

Any time you suspect that someone is trying to create a metaphorical smoke screen, mentally visualize the situation at your Pineal Gland with the Smoke Archetype over it. Look through the smoke to find the reality of the situation versus your perceived reality.

Smoke can be a form of communication. The Ancient Chinese, Ancient Greeks and indigenous peoples worldwide used smoke for quick and effective communication over long distances.

Smoke is an extremely interesting frequency, so if you choose to explore it using the Smoke Archetype, you might learn some fascinating information.

In addition, when you dream of smoke, place the scene at your Pineal Gland with the Smoke Archetype over it to find out exactly what the smoke of your dreams is communicating to you.

Water

Represents the oceans of life; emotions without boundaries; what is flowing correctly and incorrectly; cleansing; aids in Dream Interpretation.

Affirmations

The ocean of life easily provides all that I need.

I easily identify what is flowing correctly in my life.

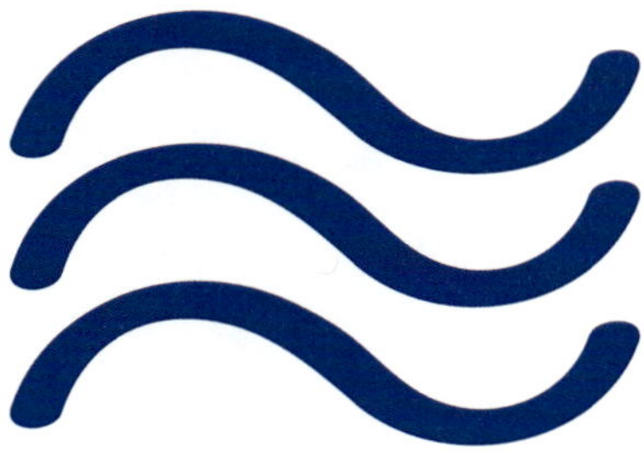

Use the Water Archetype to explore and understand the waters of the Earth. Place the Water Archetype at your Pineal Gland as you visualize various bodies of water to understand the correlation to Self.

You can also use it to understand the flow of water over the Earth, including the tides, what is above and below, weather patterns, and much more. You can be extremely creative in how you use the Water Archetype to communicate with Water in the same way the indigenous peoples do.

When you dream of water, place the dream scene at your Pineal Gland and then place the Water Archetype over it so that you can more easily understand the dream symbolism and what specific message from your superconscious mind that it conveys to you.

Part IV

Combining Archetypes

Stacking Archetypes & Creating Simple Archetype Sentences

You can stack archetypes or you can create simple archetype sentences as a boost to all of your mental work. If you have one of our specially designed Radionics boxes, you will find this process enhances whatever you want to send to your intended target.

You can stack two archetypes or more, but be careful not to do too much at one time, as this may stir up hidden undercurrents that can appear quite chaotic on their way out or their way in, depending upon what is happening.

Use three archetypes to manifest the nonphysical, such as thoughts, emotions, spirituality, intuition, and communication.

Use four archetypes to manifest into the physical, such as wealth, prosperity, family, relationships, preganancy, rejuvenation, and physical healing.

You can create your own or use the combinations on the following pages to get started.

Deprogramming

Self-Integration + Emotional Balance + Oversoul

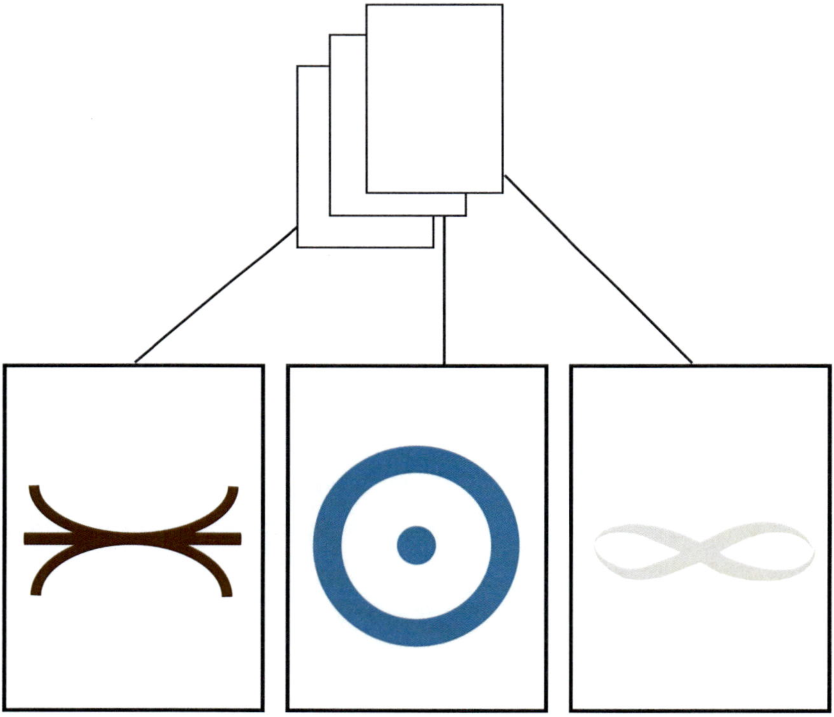

Self-integration brings Emotional Balance via the Oversoul level.

Self-Integration + Ultimate Protection + Oversoul

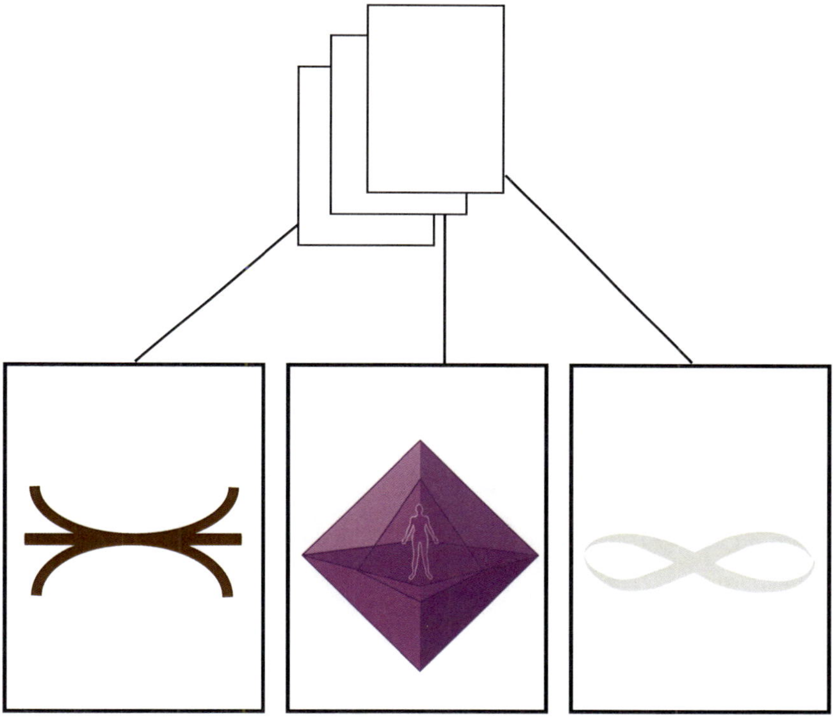

Self-integration is protected via the Oversoul level.

Self-Integration + Mental Balance + Oversoul

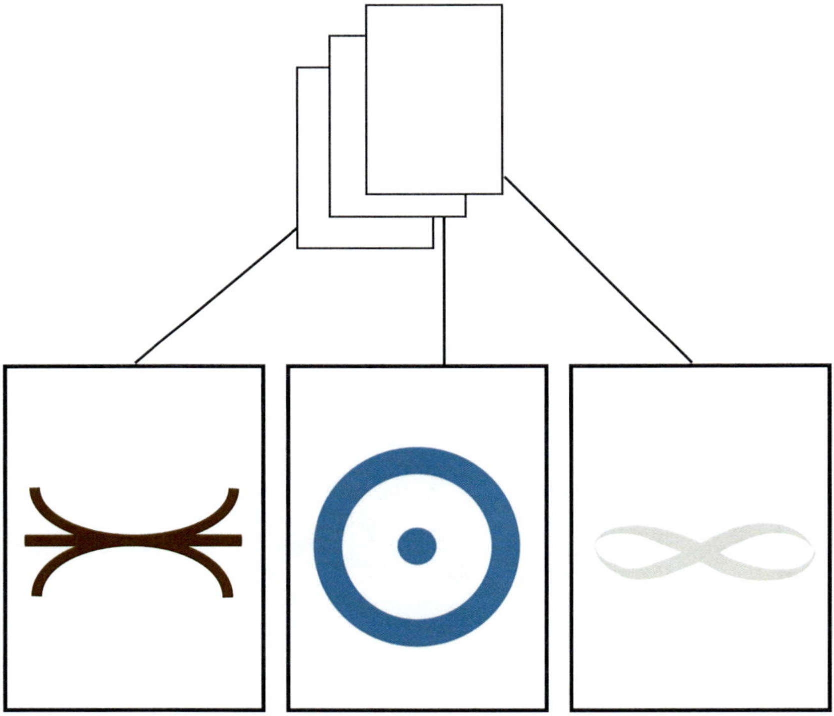

Self-integration brings mental balance via the Oversoul level.

Self-Integration + Oversoul + God-Mind

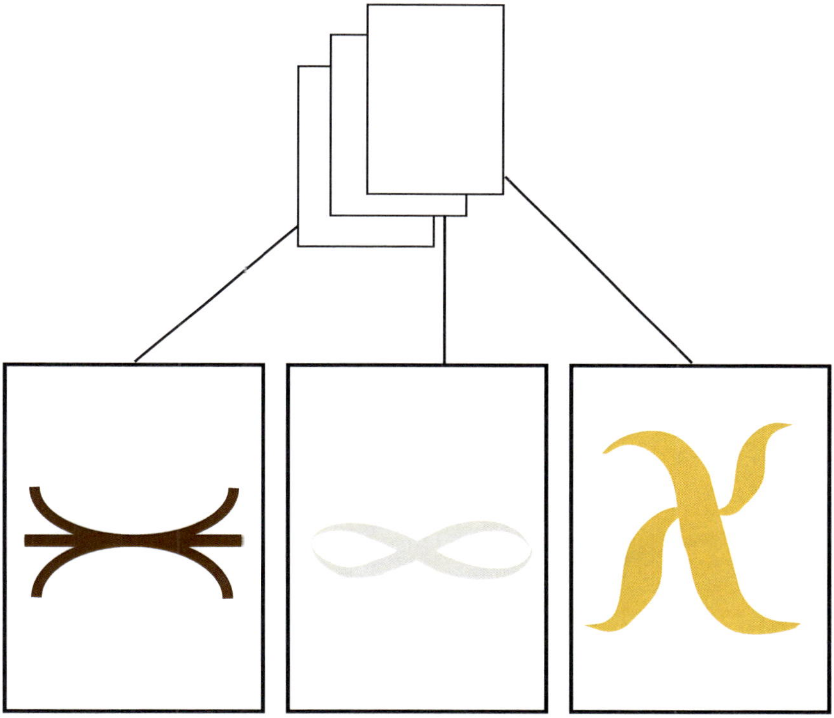

Self-integration via Oversoul and God-Mind levels.

Self-Integration + Happiness + Ultimate Protection

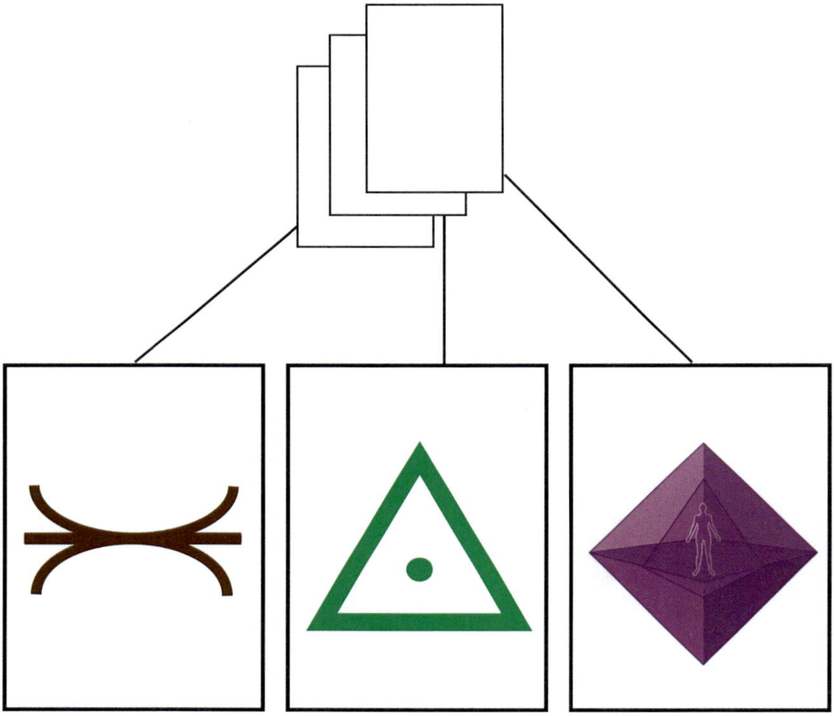

Self-integration brings Happiness that is Protected.

Self-Integration + Power + Perfect Manifestation/Creation

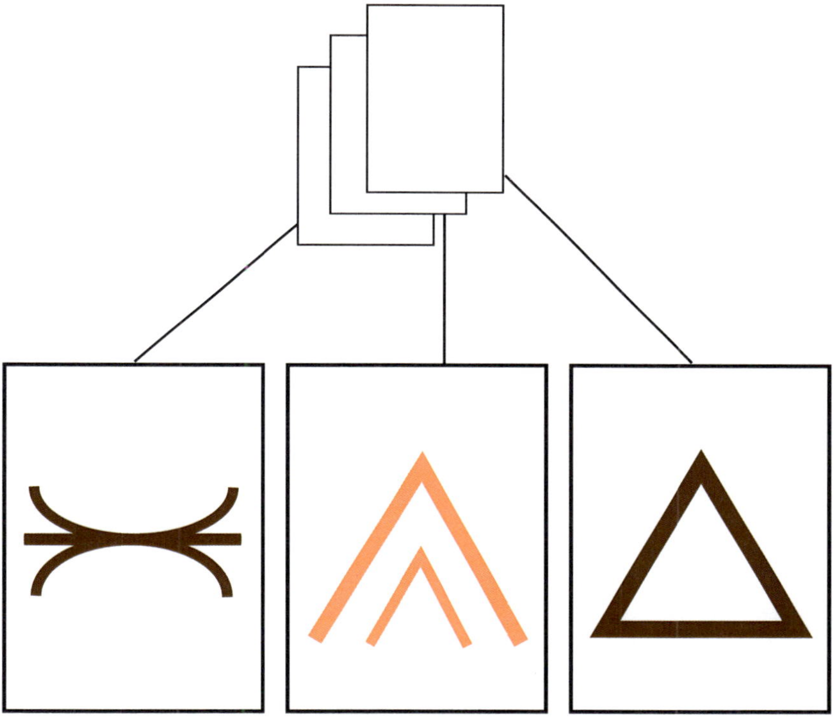

Self-integration is Powerfully and Perfectly Manifests/Creates.

Health, Emotional & Mental

Overall Healing + New Beginnings + Happiness

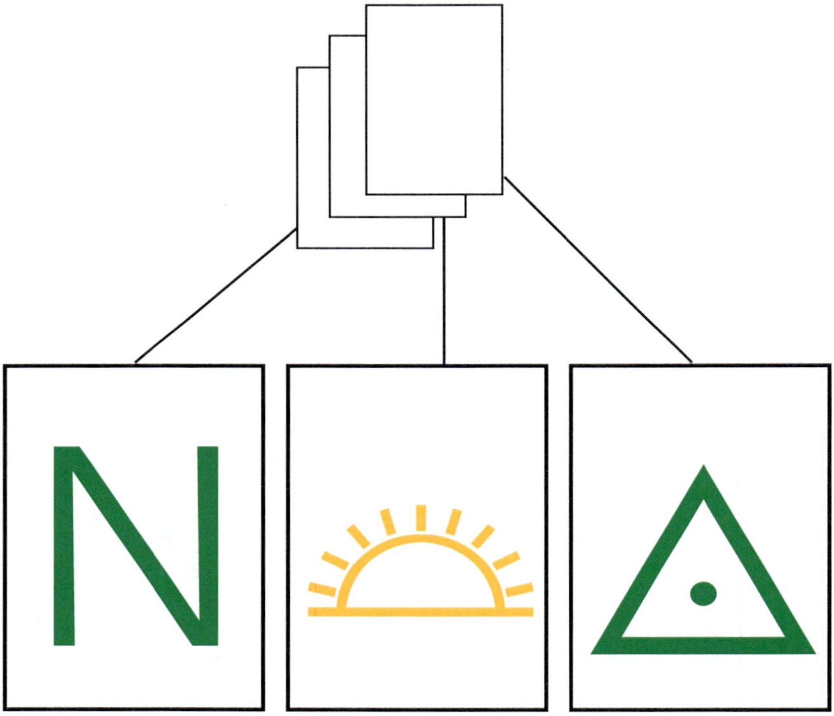

Overall Healing brings New Beginnings in Happiness.

Overall Healing + Emotional Balance + Mental Balance

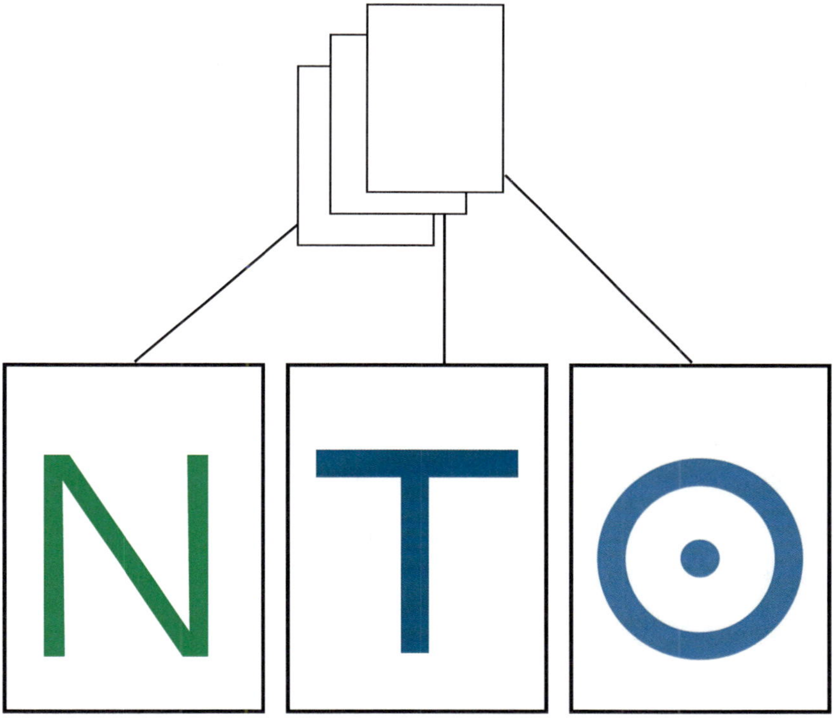

Overall Healing brings Emotional Balance and Mental Balance.

Overall Healing + Releases & Resolves Past Issues + Self-Integration

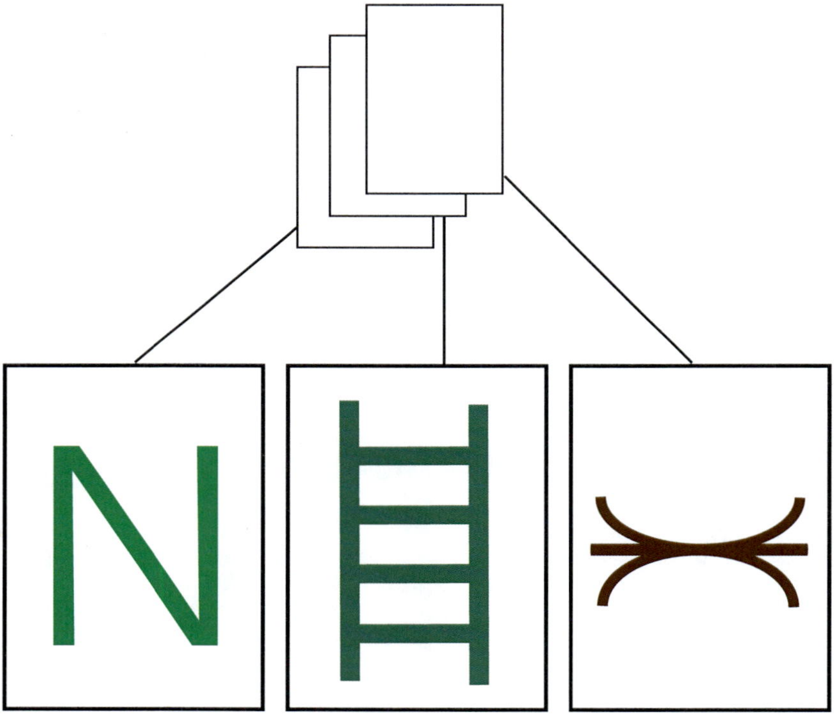

Overall Healing Releases and Resolves Past Issue that allows for Self-Integration.

Overall Healing + Wolf Frequency + Ultimate Protection

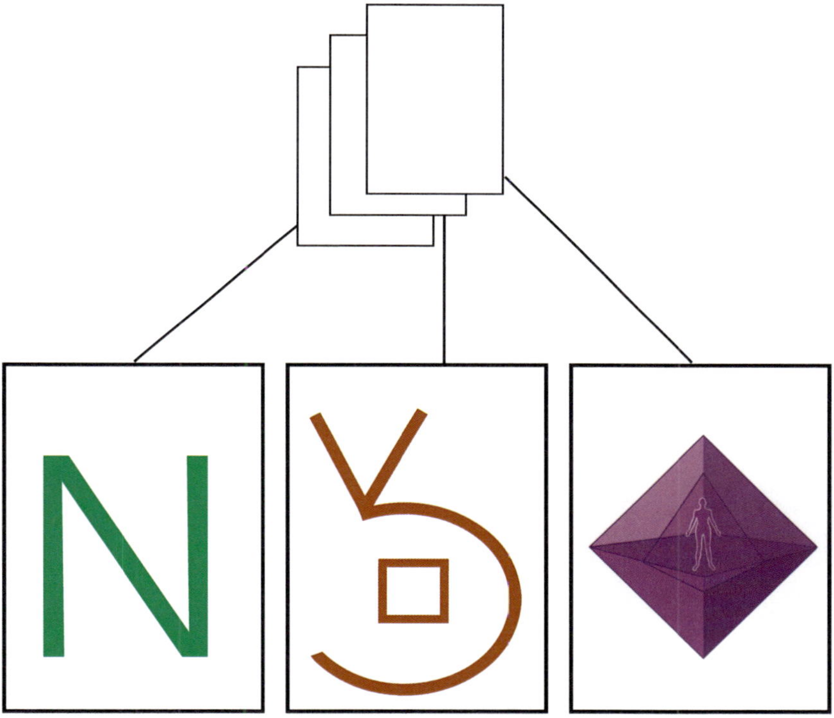

Overall Healing in family relationships is protected.

Overall Healing + Communication + Happiness

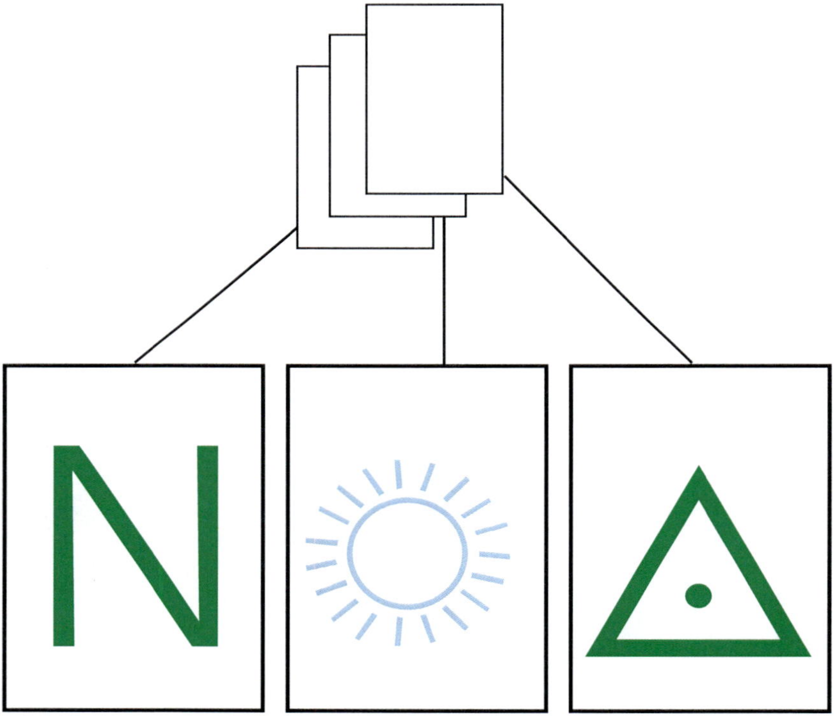

Overall Healing in Communication brings Happiness.

Overall Healing + Dolphin Frequency + Oversoul

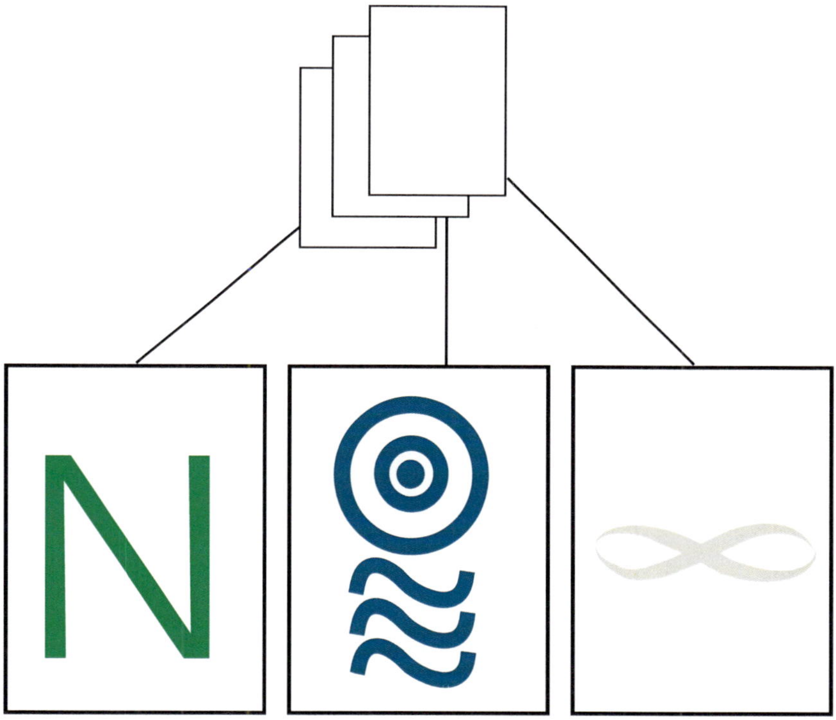

Overall Healing using Dolphin Frequency connects to Oversoul level.

Health, Physical

Overall Healing + Chakra System +
Perfect Manifestation/Creation + Expansion

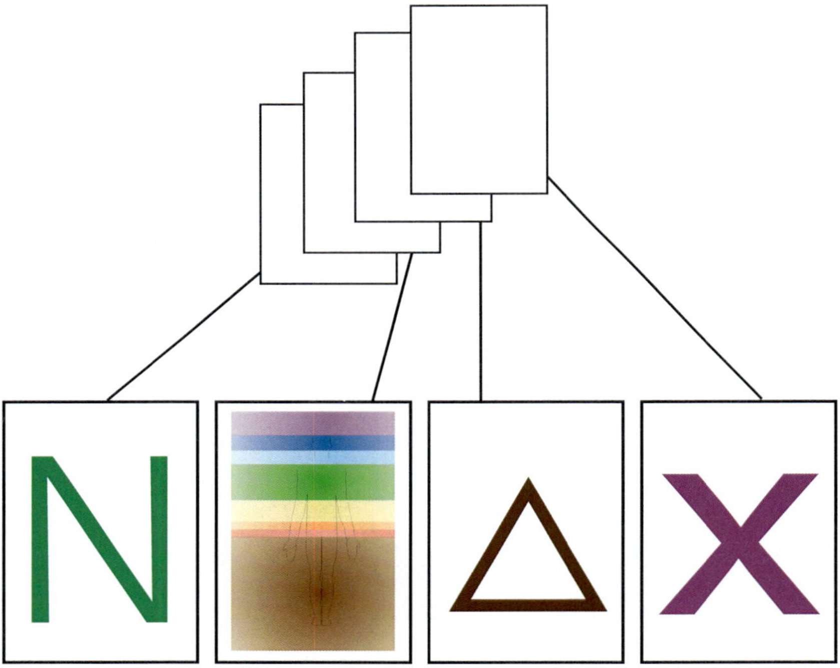

Overall Healing to the Chakra System Perfectly Manifests/ Creates and Expands.

Overall Healing + Green Psychic Flush + Rejuvenation + Expansion

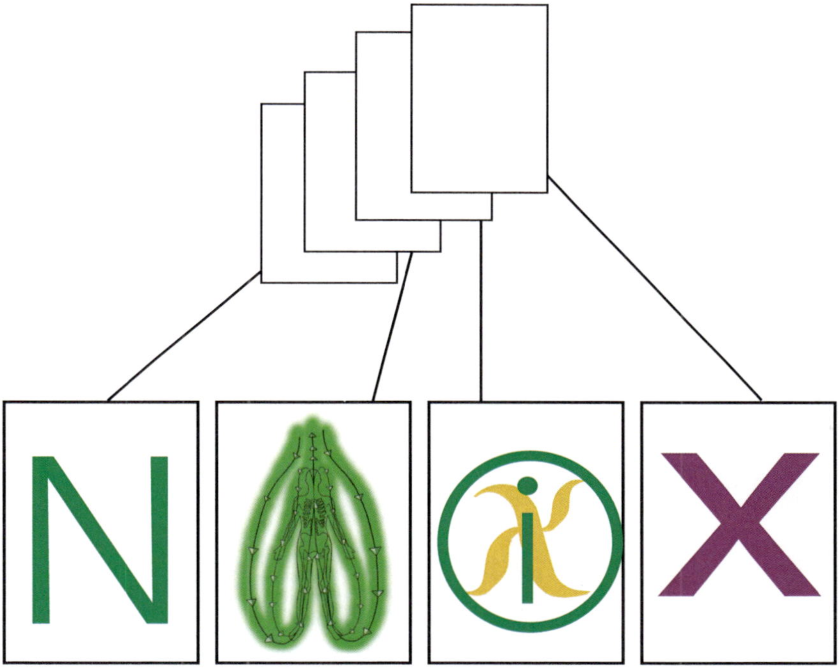

Overall Healing to the Psychic energy system Rejuvenates and Expands.

Overall Healing + Chakra System + Green Psychic Flush + Ultimate Protection

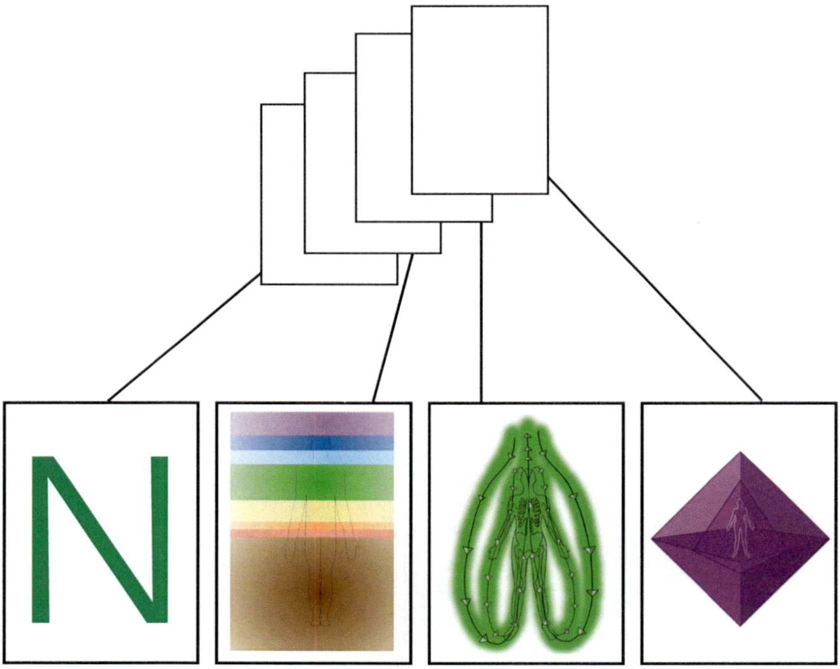

Overall Healing to the Chakra System and Psychic energy system is Protected.

Overall Healing + Green Psychic Flush + Perfect Manifestastion/Creation + Expansion

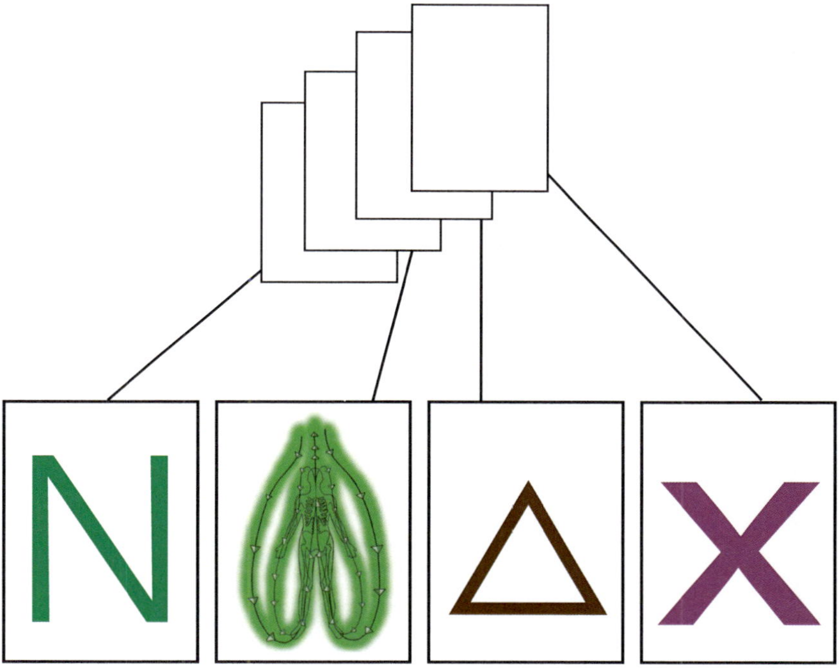

Overall Healing to the Psychic energy system Perfectly Manifests/ Creates and Expands.

Overall Healing + Release & Resolve Past Issues + Self-Integration + Ultimate Protection

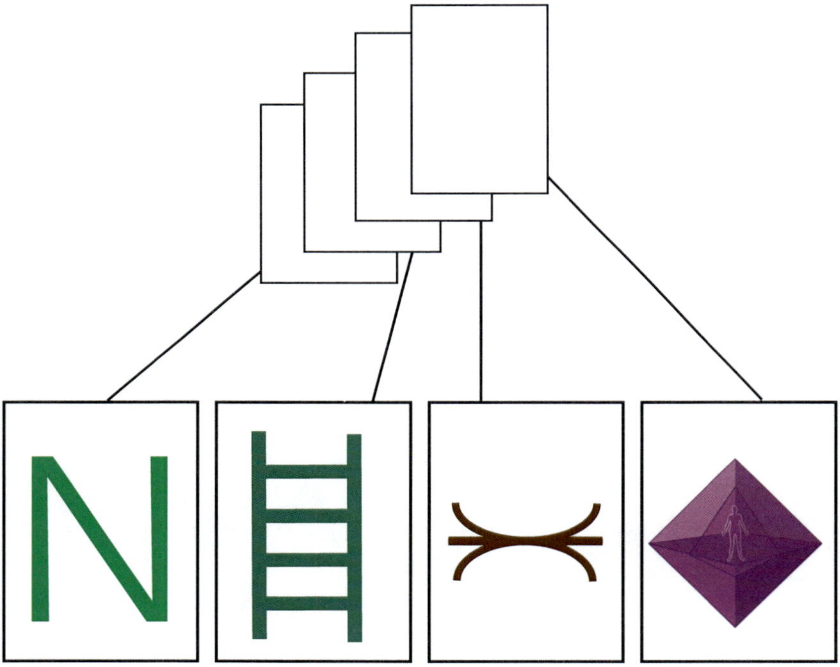

Overall Healing Releases and Resolves Past Issues and allows Self-Integration, which is all Protected.

Overall Healing + Bear Frequency +
Mental Balance + Emotional Balance

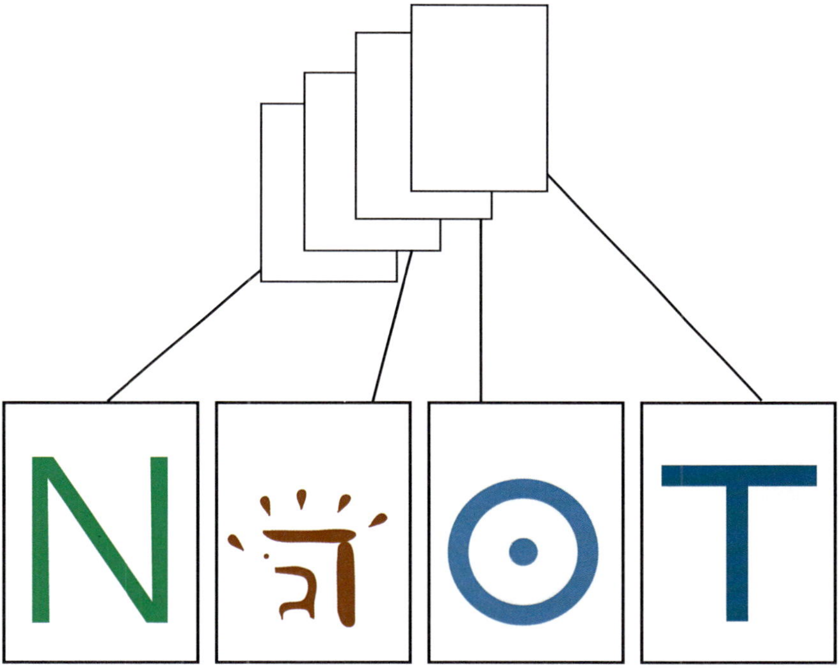

Overall Healing goes within to create
Mental and Emotional Balance.

**Overall Healing + Chakra System +
Logos Christos + Lion Frequency**

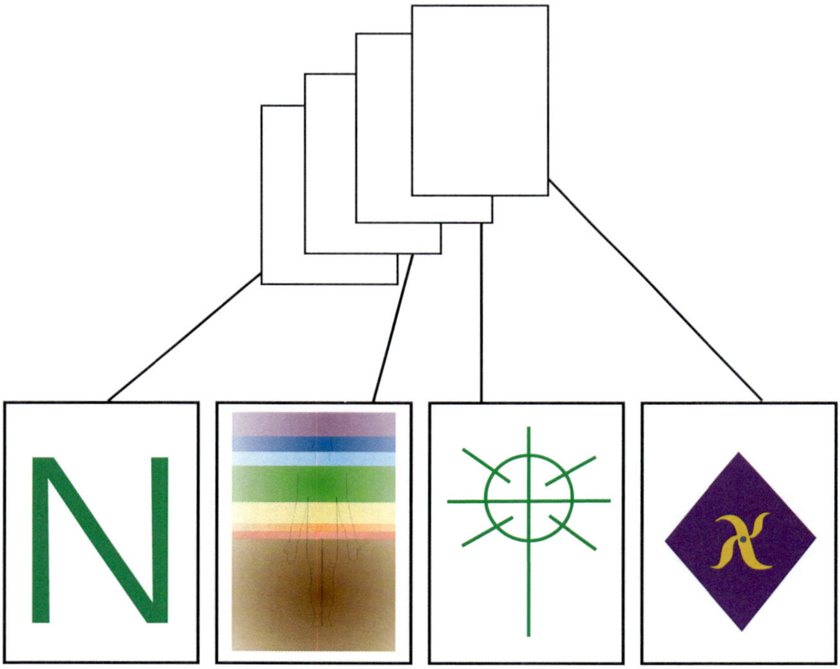

Overall Healing in the Chakra System is enhanced and connected to the highest frequency between physical and nonphysical.

Relationships

Relationships + Wolf Frequency + Ultimate Protection

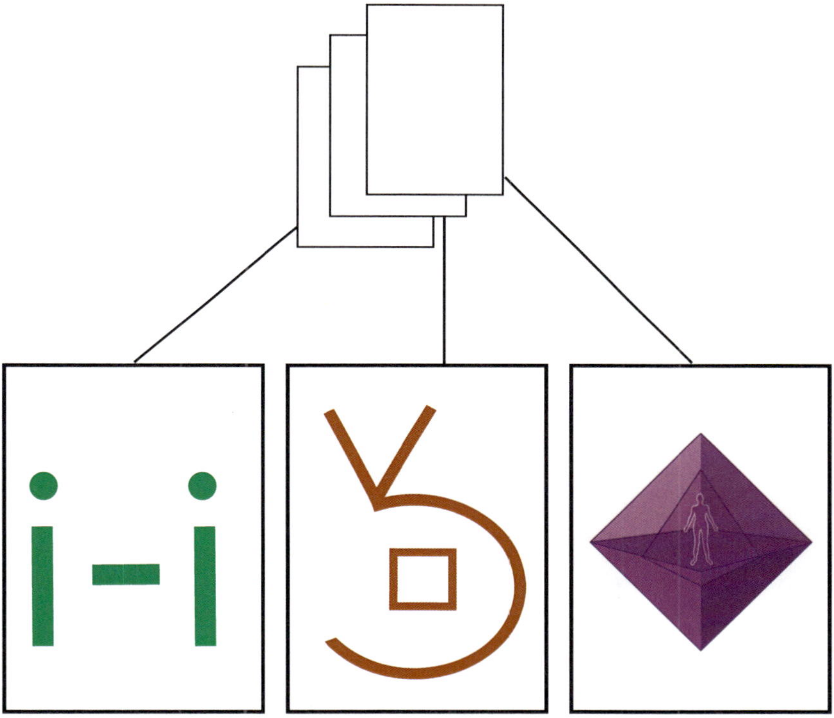

Relationships that are family are Protected.

Relationships + New Beginnings + Happiness

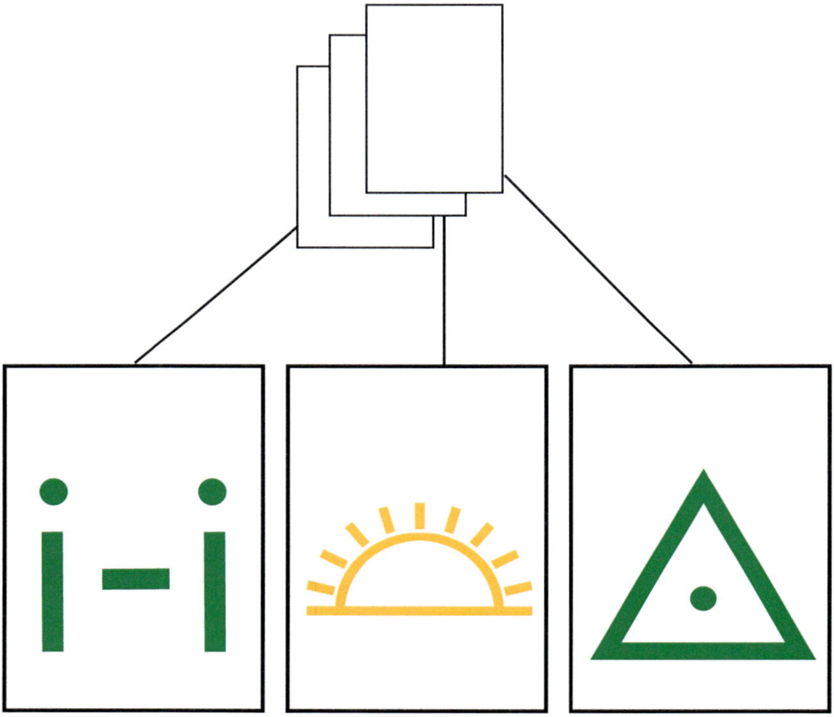

Relationships have New Beginnings that bring Happiness.

Relationships + Resolve & Release Old Issues + Power

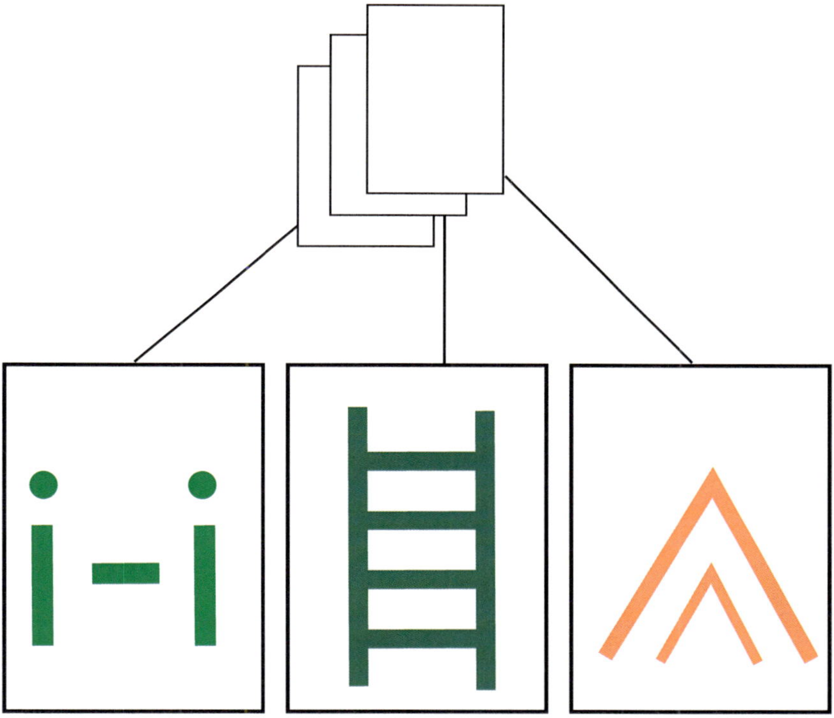

Relationships Resolve and Release Old Issues Powerfully.

Relationships + Communication + Overall Healing

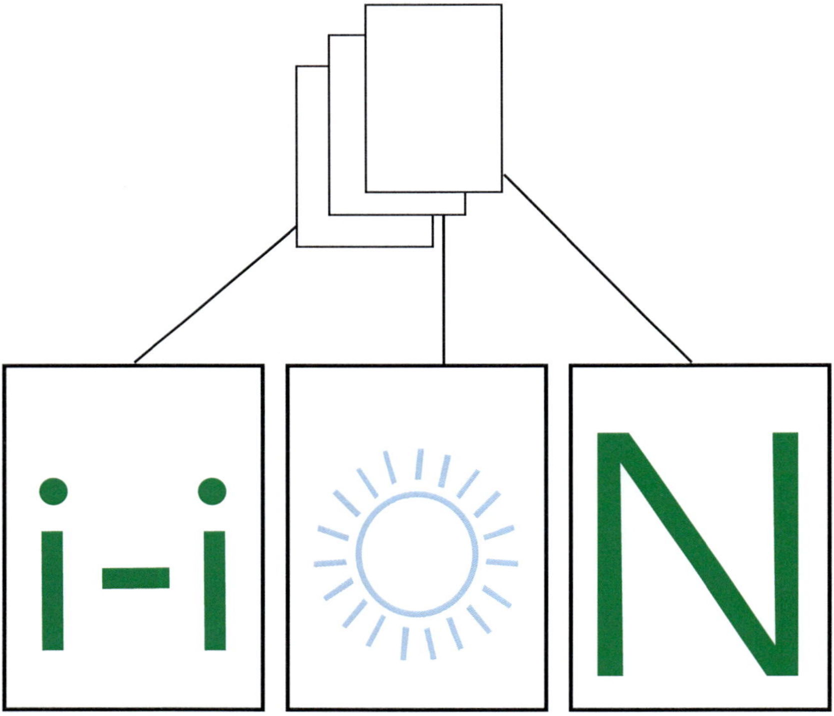

Relationships Communicate for Overall Healing.

Relationships + Male Orgasm + Female Orgasm + Pregnancy

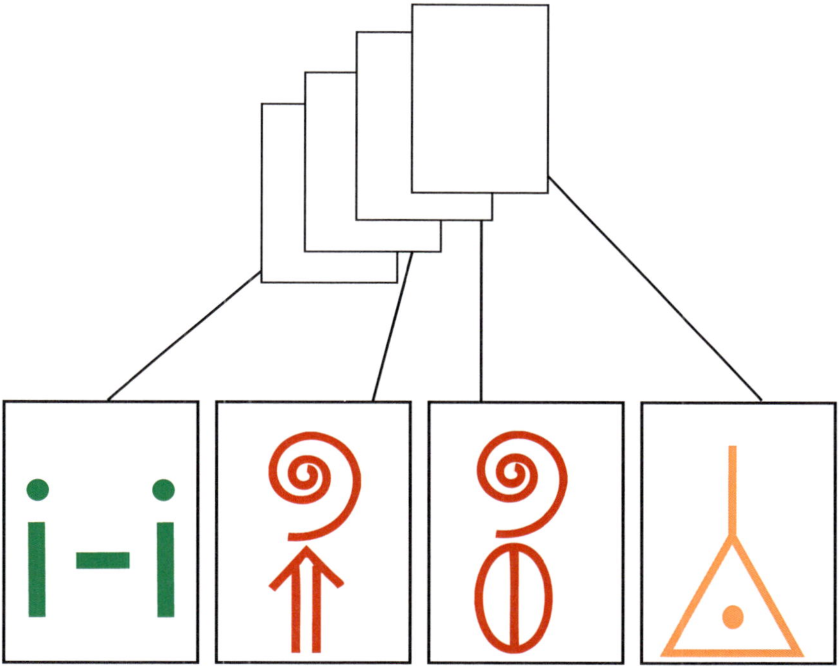

Relationships aid Male virility and Female responsiveness to create a Pregnancy.

Relationships + Spiritual & Intuition Connection + Expansion

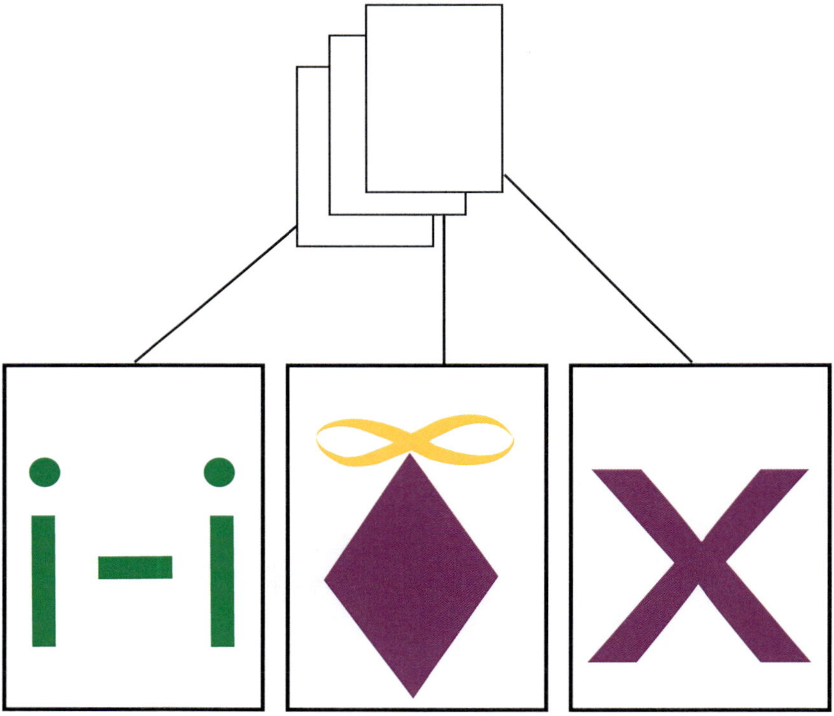

Relationships with Spiritual and Intuition Connections Expand.

Spiritual

Spiritual & Intuition Connection + Communication + Oversoul

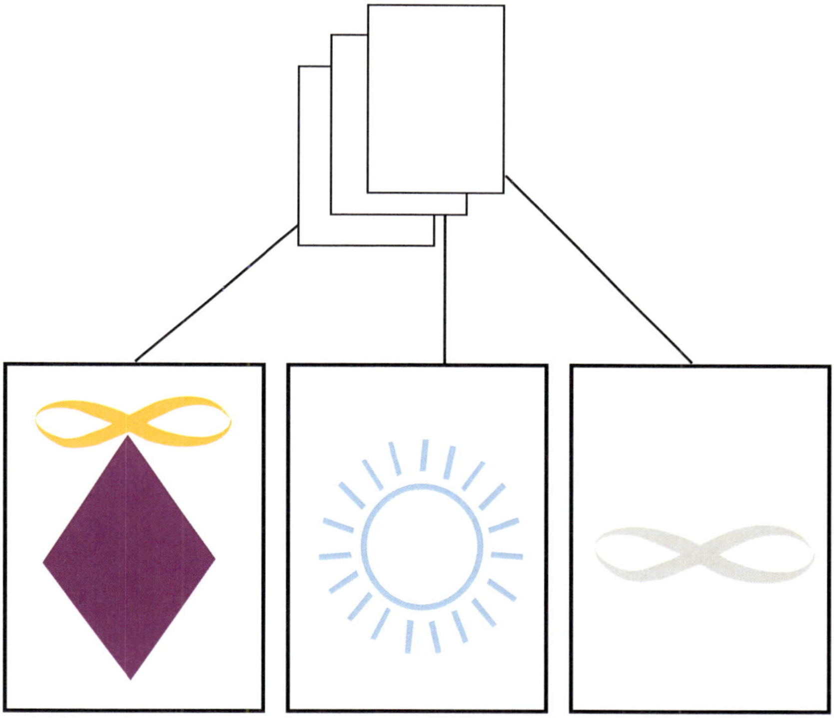

Spiritual and Intuition Connections aid Communication to Oversoul.

Spiritual & Intuition Connection + Release & Resolve Past Issues + Happiness

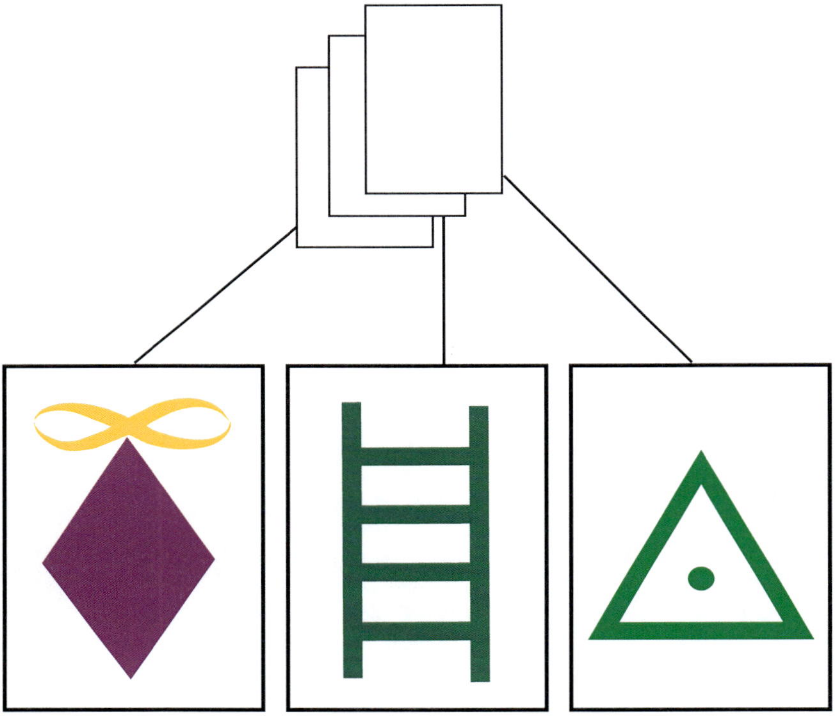

Spiritual and Intuition Connection Releases and Resolves Past Issues to create Happiness.

Spiritual & Intuition Connection + Bear Frequency + Release & Resolve Past Issues

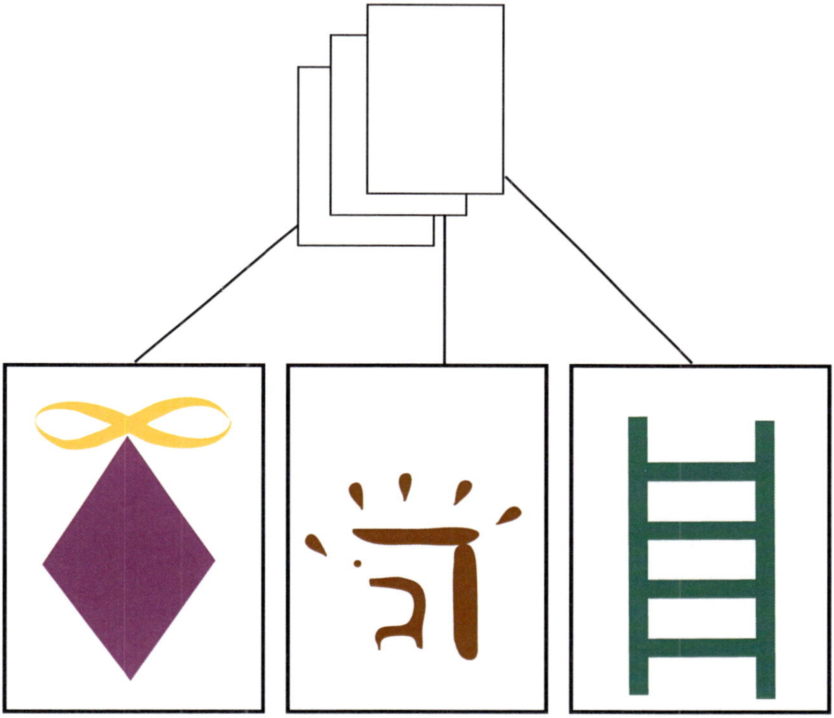

Spiritual and Intuition Connections go within to Release and Resolve Past Issues.

Spiritual & Intuition Connection + New Beginnings + God-Mind

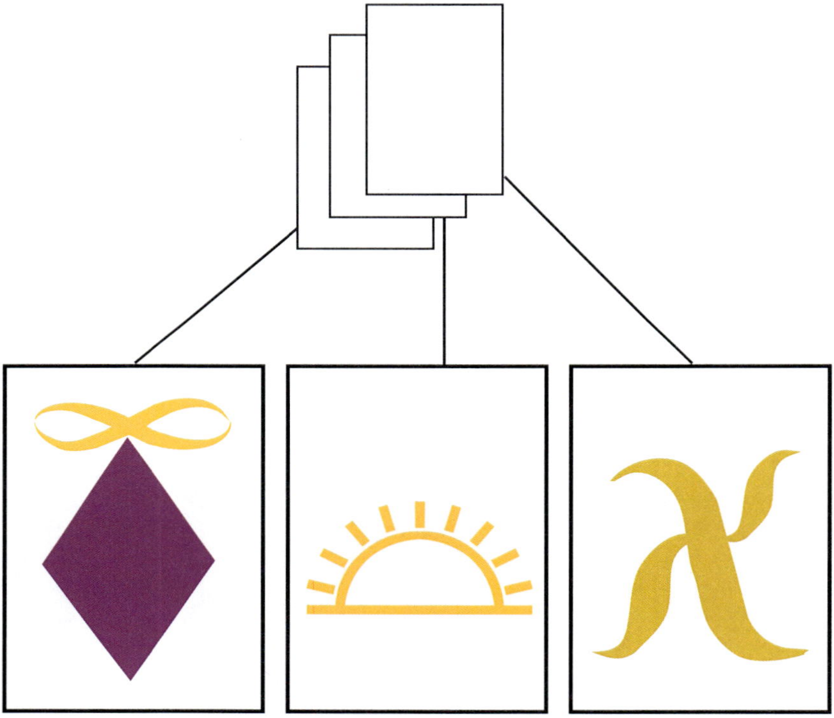

Spiritual and Intuition Connections enhance New Beginnings with God-Mind.

Spiritual & Intuition Connection + Expansion + Oversoul

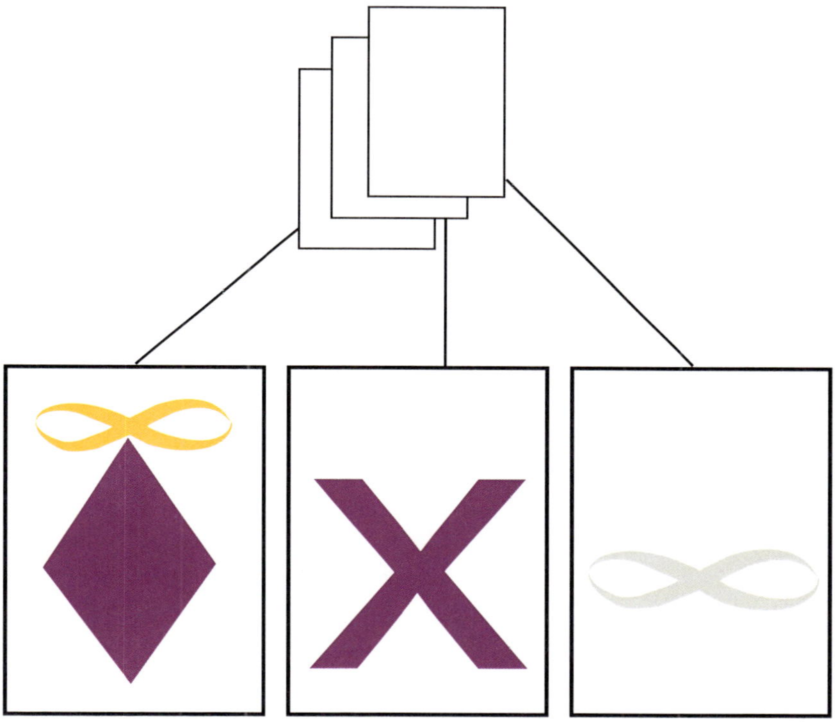

Spiritual and Intuition Connections Expand into Oversoul.

Spiritual & Intuition Connection + Wisdom + God-Mind

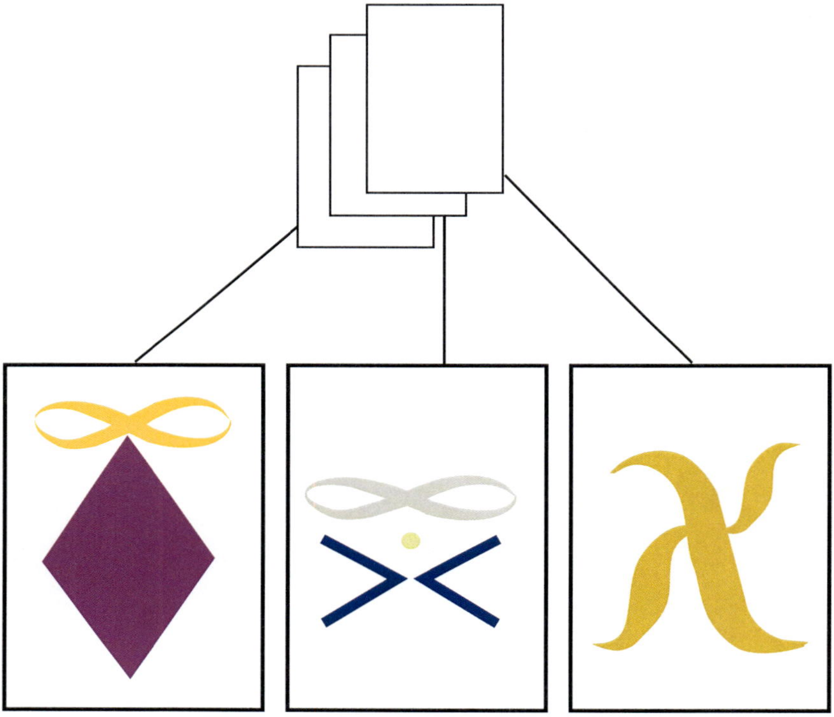

Spiritual and Intuition Connection aid in attaining Wisdom from God-Mind.

Spiritual & Intuition Connection + Leadership + Individualized Consciousness

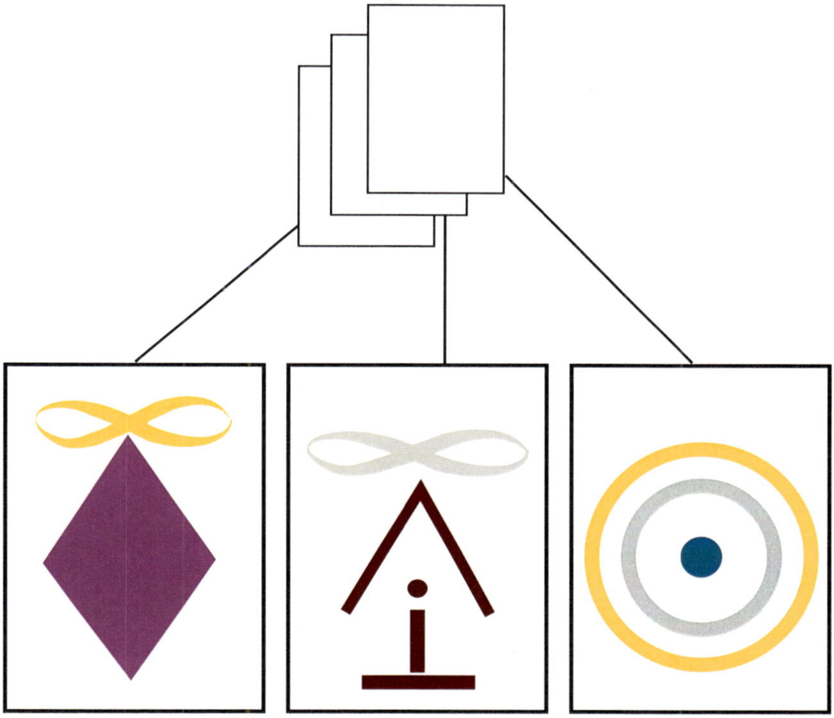

Spiritual and Intuition Connections aid Leadership into Individualized Consciousness.

Spiritual & Intuition Connection + Lion Frequency + God-Mind

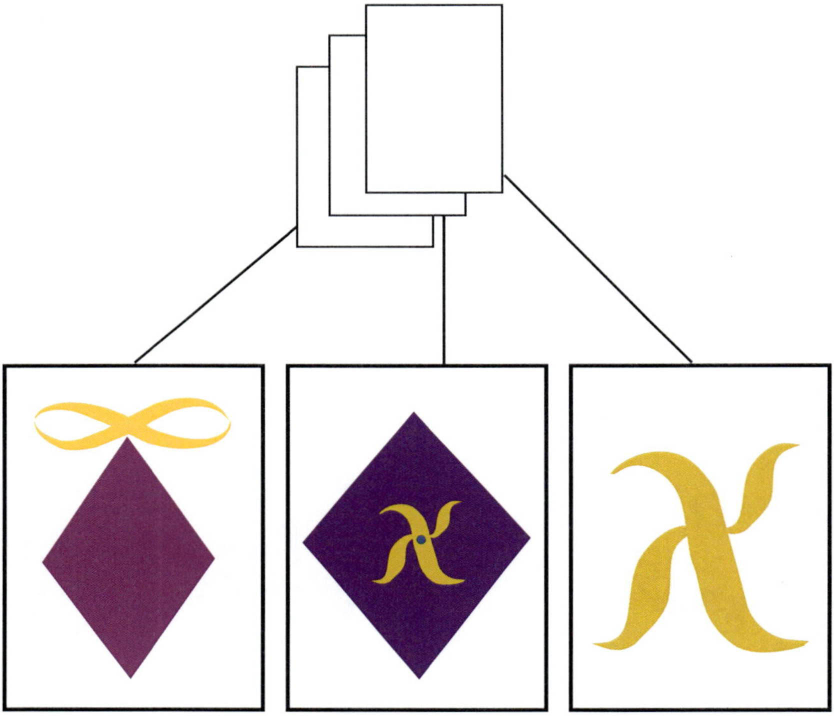

Spiritual and Intuition Connection is enhanced with direct awareness to God-Mind.

Wealth

Wealth & Prosperity + Spiritual & Intuition Connection + Wisdom + Perfect Manifestation/Creation

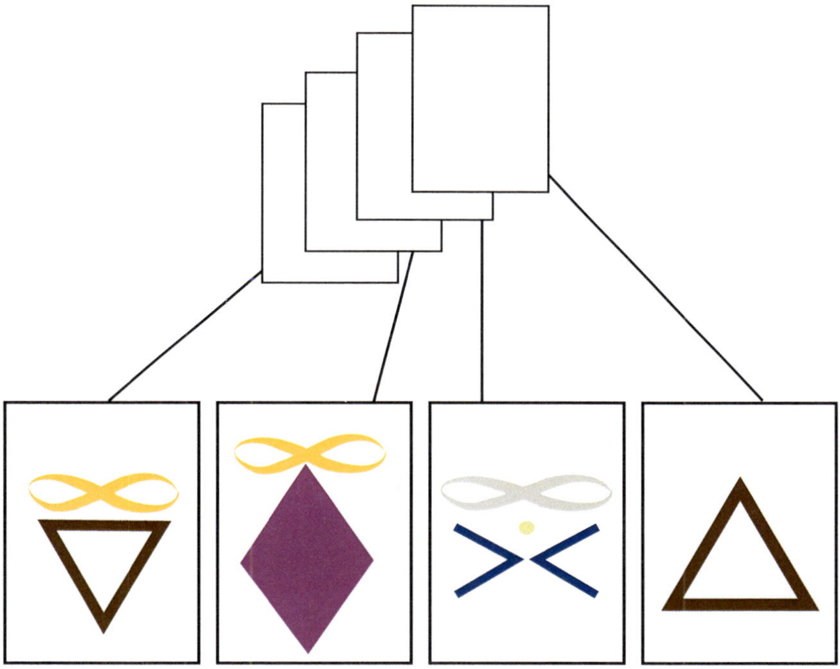

Wealth and Prosperity are enhanced via Spiritual and Intuition Connections as well as Wisdom for Perfect Manifestation and Creation.

Wealth & Prosperity + Power + Expansion + Ultimate Protection

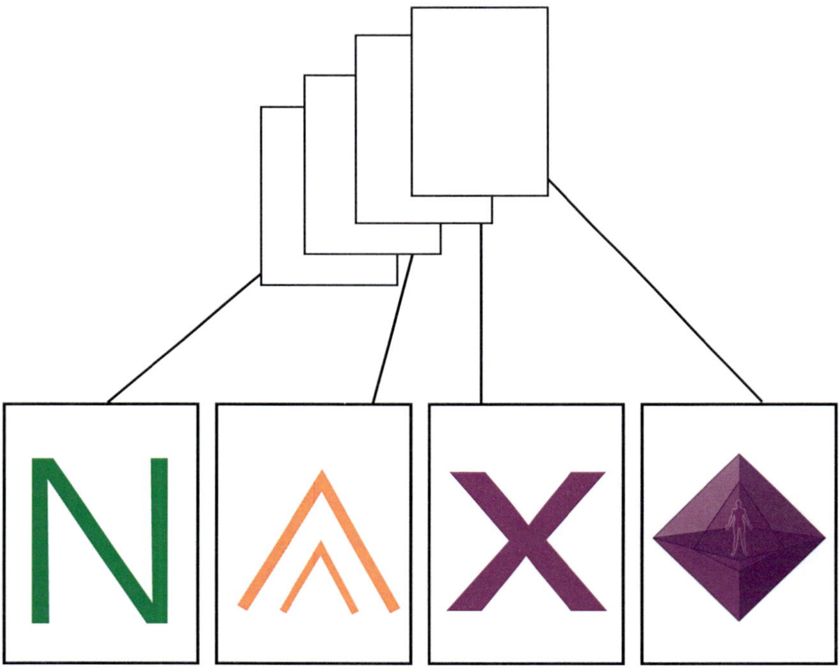

Wealth and Prosperity Powerfully Expand with Protection.

Wealth & Prosperity + New Beginnings + Happiness + Perfect Manifestation/Creation

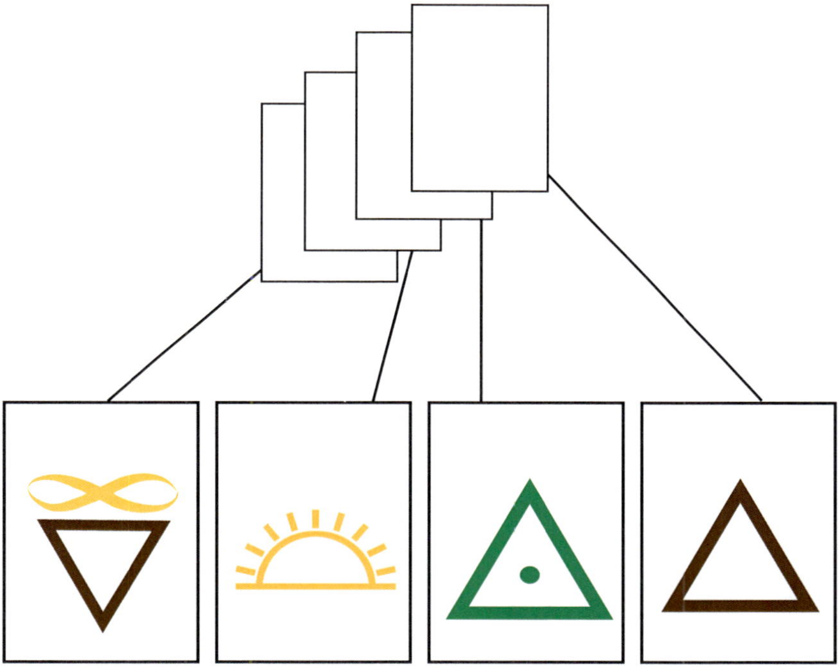

Wealth and Prosperity have New Beginnings that bring Happiness into Perfect Manifestation and Creation.

Wealth & Prosperity + Power + New Beginnings + Expansion

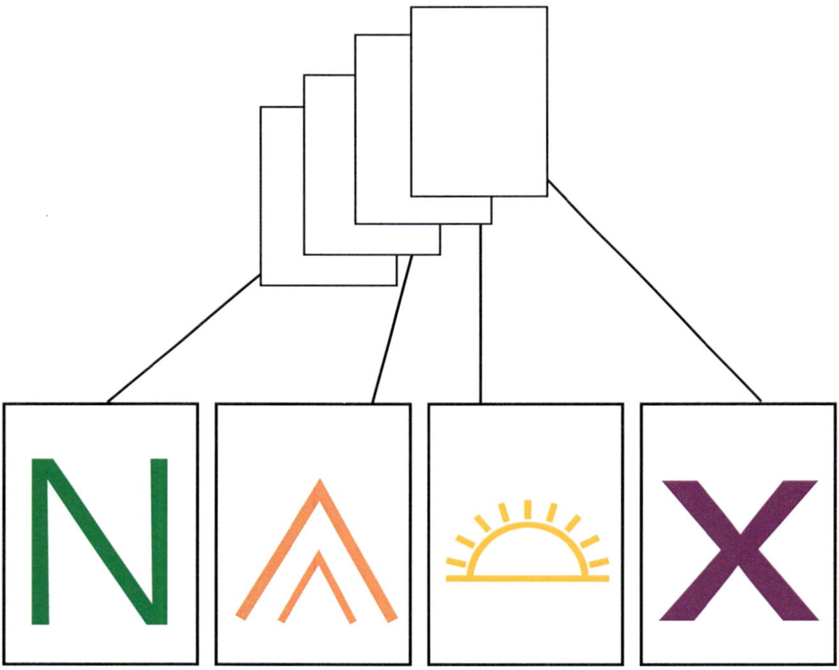

Wealth and Prosperity have Powerful New Beginnings that Expand.

Wealth & Prosperity + Overall Healing + Oversoul + God-Mind

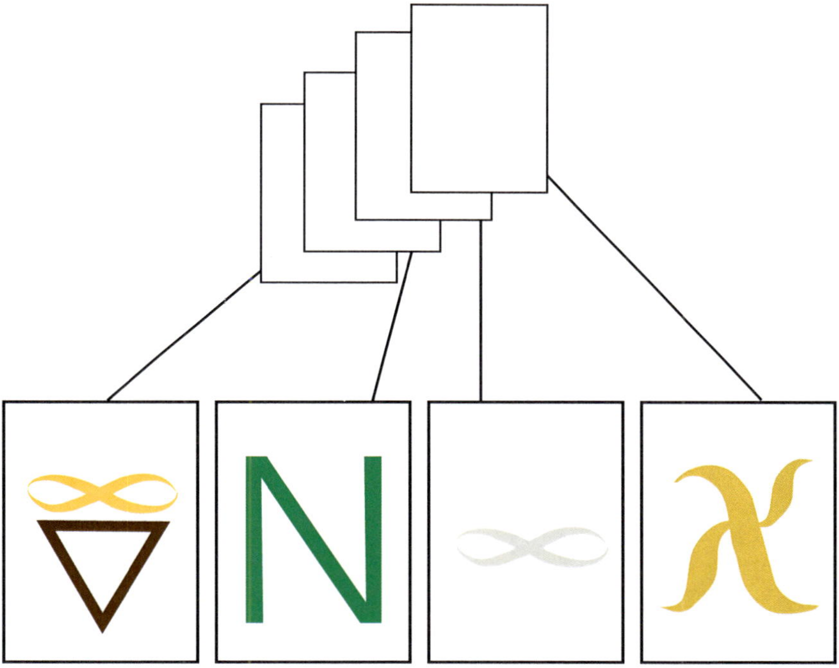

Wealth and Prosperity Heals with the aid of Oversoul and God-Mind.

Wealth & Prosperity + Merge with Aspects of Alternate Selves in Other Realities + Ultimate Protection + Lion Frequency

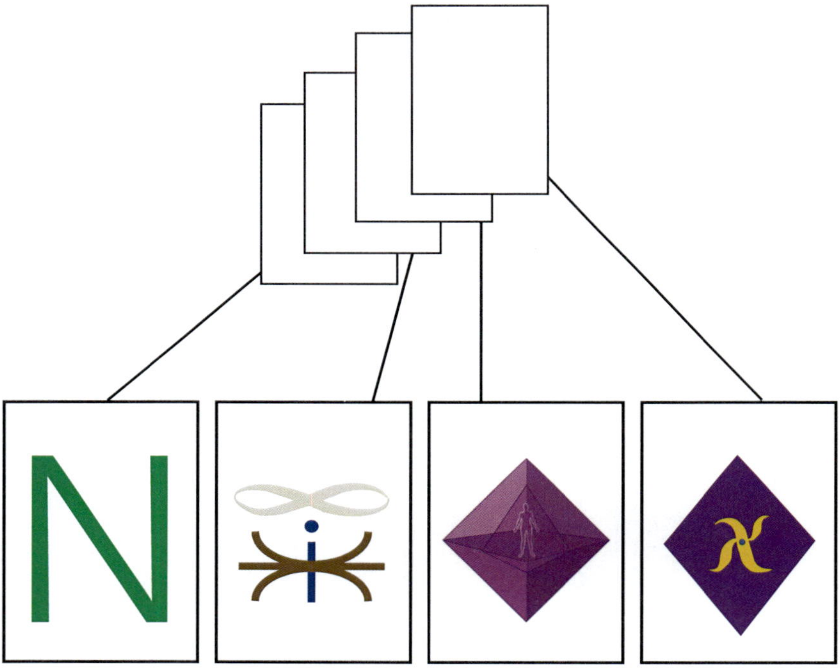

Wealth and Prosperity Merges with Aspects of Alternative Selves in Other Realities Connected and Protected via Lion Frequency.

Part V

Complex Archetypes for Higher Frequencies

White Winged Dragon Complex Archetype

Use the White Winged Dragon Complex Archetype first until you are comfortable with the frequency.

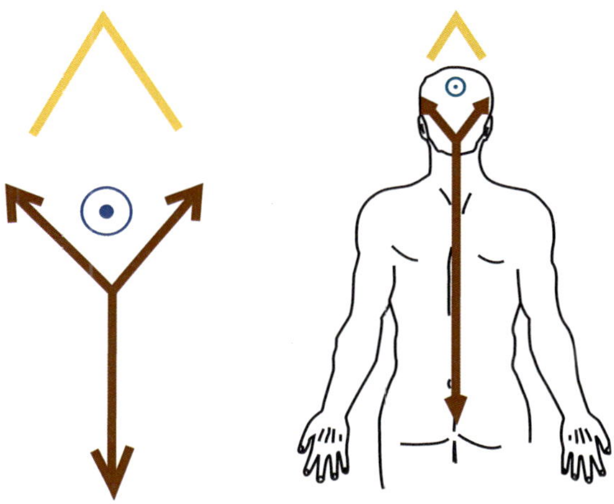

Archetype Placement

Place the brown arrowed-Y shape on the spinal column with the left top arrow in your left brain, the right top arrow in your right brain, and the bottom arrow at the coccyx bone. The royal blue circle and dot are at the pineal gland at the center of the head. The inverted gold "V" is over the crown of the head.

Archetype Use

This complex archetype helps you access the White Winged Dragon Frequency.

In this frequency, you are able to access the foundational levels of your core personality as a segment of God-Mind. This frequency enables you to manifest on the physical Earth plane from the highest levels of the nonphysical. Use the White Winged Dragon Frequency when you want to create from the deepest core of yourself.

White Winged Lion Complex Archetype

Use the White Winged Lion Complex Archetype after you are comfortable with the White Winged Dragon Complex Archetype. Use the White Winged Lion Complex Archetype until you are comfortable with the frequency.

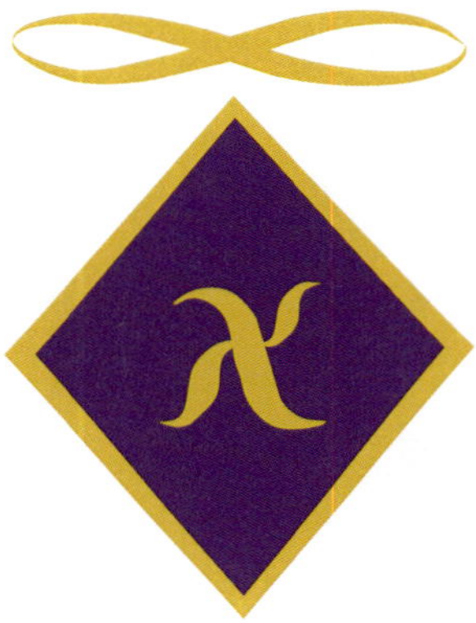

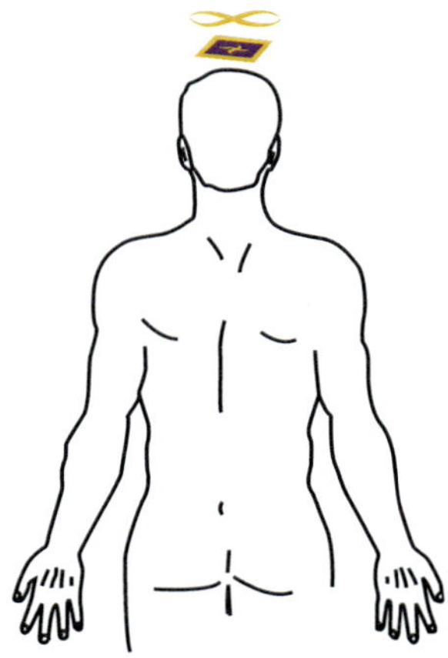

Archetype Placement

Place the gold-outlined purple diamond as a platform lying flat on the crown of the head. The Gold Aleph stands up on the middle of the diamond platform facing forward. The Aleph and the platform are perpendicular to each other. The Gold Infinity Symbol is above the Gold Aleph facing forward.

Archetype Use

This complex archetype connects you to the White Winged Lion Frequency. This is the highest level of Lion Frequency that connects directly to God-Mind, which allows you to feel and use that energy. The White Winged Lion Frequency allows you to create anything that you have in your mind, so be careful what you think about while in this frequency.

White Winged Dragon & White Winged Lion Merging

After you feel comfortable separately using the White Winged Dragon Complex Archetype and the White Winged Lion Complex Archetype, then you are ready to merge these two complex archetypes together.

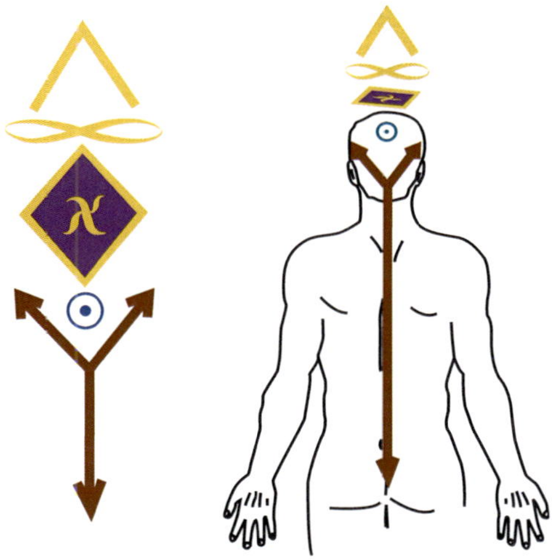

Archetype Placement

Place the complex archetypes as shown. In addition, place three Brown Merger Archetypes as follows:

1. Pineal Gland
2. Brain Stem
3. Heart Chakra

Archetype Use

This ultimate frequency connects to all of your interdimensional selves in all areas of existence. Mentally direct what aspects of Self you wish to pull in. For example:

I now merge with all my alternate selves in every reality where I exist that are in conscious communication with my Oversoul and God-Mind.

I now merge with all my alternate selves in every reality where I exist with exceptional mental and physical health.

I now merge with all my alternate selves in every reality where I exist with fabulous relationships.

I now merge with all my alternate selves in every reality where I exist that are not programmed.

I now merge with all my alternate selves in every reality where I exist in opulent wealth.

The merging of the Reptilian Frequency and Mammalian Frequency that comprise humanity allows you to end the innate human struggle started by the Original Experiment, which merged Reptilian and Mammalian genetics to create humankind. Ending the struggle allows you to more comfortably and easily achieve all goals.

Sea Serpent

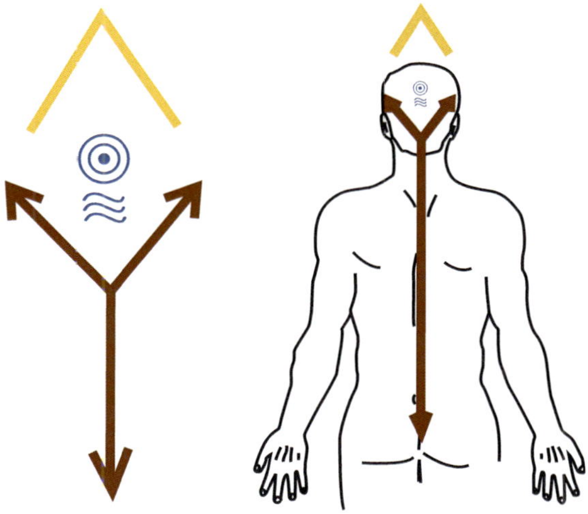

Archetype Placement

Place the brown arrowed-Y shape on the spinal column with the left top arrow in your left brain, the right top arrow in your right brain, and the bottom arrow at the coccyx bone. The royal blue circle and dot are at the pineal gland at the center of the head. The addition of the three wavy royal blue lines adds the entry code to Dolphin Frequency. The inverted Gold "V" is over the crown of the head.

Archetype Use

Use this complex archetype anytime for additional exploration under the oceans or under any large body of water to further understand the emotional depths of Self.

Part VI

Extras

What is Your T-Bar?

Your brain is divided into two halves, the left and right hemispheres. Logic and Physical Reality thoughts are centered in your left brain. Spirituality, creativity and emotional thoughts are centered in your right brain.

Your pineal gland is located between the two halves of your brain, creating balance. Your pineal gland projects an archetype into depending upon your genetics. This archetype is one of these three:

Ankh

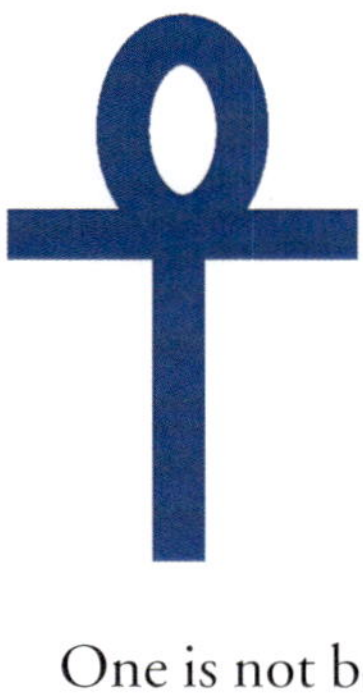

Upper case "T"

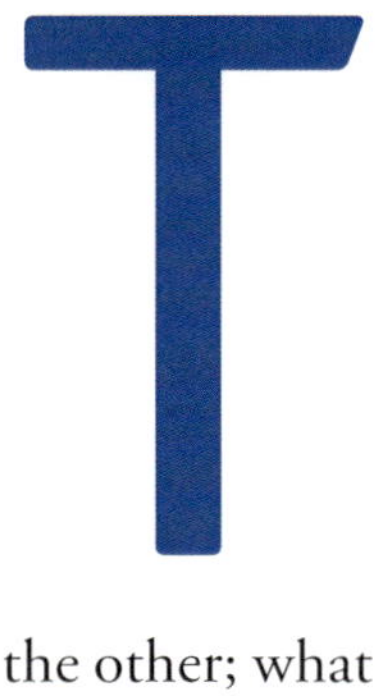

Lower case "t"

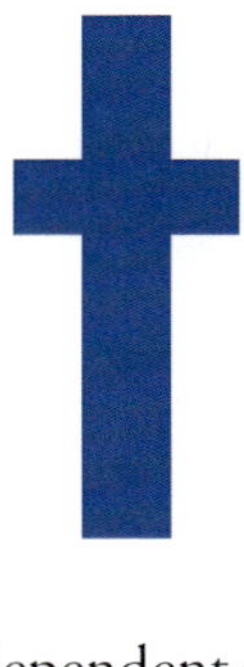

One is not better than the other; what is projected is dependent entirely upon your genetics. Some people often see more than one T-Bar or they notice that their T-Bar Archetype changes. This is because you may have more than one set of genetic codes active, or your genetic codes can open and close, depending upon what is going on in your life.

Be sure to keep your T-Bar Archetype balanced at all times so that the arms of the "T" are always perpendicular to the Earth. This keeps your emotions and mind balanced and grounded, making your life much easier for you.

If you cannot determine your T-Bar Archetype, you can always use the archetype for the Pineal Gland, which is:

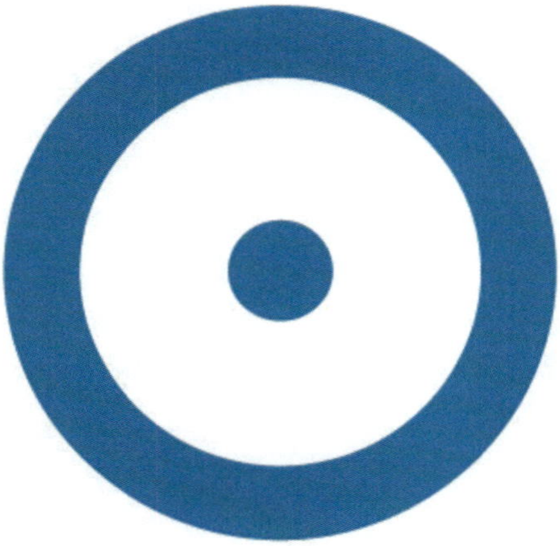

What is Your Chakra System?

Chakra Spinning

Every living human being has a chakra system. The word "chakra" is a Hindu/Sanskrit word that means "wheel," referring to the way chakras spin within the energy system of the physical body.

Humans have seven main chakra centers, located from the perineum up to the crown. Each one has a specific function, color, and meaning, and corresponds to specific organs located in that part of the body.

The human chakra system is as follows:

Grounding Center

Actually, this is not a chakra at all, but rather the Earth's magnetic field connecting to the body. This extends from the feet to the perineum. The color here is brown.

Root Chakra

This is located at the perineum and extends to the top of the pubic bone. The color here is pale red.

Sacral Chakra

This chakra is located between the top of the pubic bone and the navel. The color here is pale orange.

Solar Plexus Chakra

This chakra is located between the navel and the sternum. The color here is pale yellow.

Heart Chakra

This chakra is situated between the sternum and the clavicle bone. The color here is medium green.

Throat Chakra

This chakra starts at the base of the throat and extends to just below the tip of the nose. The color here is ice blue.

Pineal Chakra

This chakra is located from the tip of the nose to the middle of the forehead. The color here is royal blue.

Crown Chakra

This chakra is located at the top of the skull. The color here is violet.

It is absolutely necessary for every human being to begin the day by spinning his/her chakras.

Do it before getting out of bed in the morning. You may either spin them in a clockwise or counterclockwise motion, whichever one is better for you. Please note, however, that all chakras must be spun in the same direction each day. The only time it is advisable to reverse the spinning direction is to counter the effects of a traumatic or particularly stressful day. Do this by spinning from the top down; otherwise always spin from the bottom up.

When spinning your chakras, begin by visualizing yourself in a cylindrical tube with each of the specific colors in their respective locations. Next, visualize brown in the Grounding Center. Work your way up to the crown using the appropriate color in each chakra band. Remember to always spin all chakra bands in the same direction.

What is Your Psychic Energy?

Your Psychic Energy is your personal energy. Your physical body uses psychic energy to walk, talk, breathe, digest food, and so forth. Use this Psychic Energy Green Flush to oxygenate and work out any knots or blockages you have within your physical body.

Keeping your psychic energy flowing through your physical body helps to promote physical health and harmony.

Green Flush

Flushing the Body

Purpose: To oxygenate, regenerate, and open the flow of psychic (personal) energy.

From the top of your head, breathe in medium green from your Oversoul. Bring this color all the way down the outside of your body to the bottom of your feet. Bring this green up through the bottom of your feet, permeating every cell of your Being, flushing out all that you no longer need as it permeates the cellular structure on all levels. Feel the tingling of the energy as it moves through each section/cell of your body.

Bring the green up through your legs, torso, neck, and out through the top of your head, releasing all that you no longer need (represented by the black) out the top of your head.

Allow the green flush to continue down through your shoulders, flowing down your arms and out your fingertips, continuing to flush out all that you no longer need. Repeat the cycle as long as you feel necessary, flushing, oxygenating, regenerating and opening up your psychic energy lines as it flows, continually releasing all that you no longer need up through the top of your head up to your Oversoul.

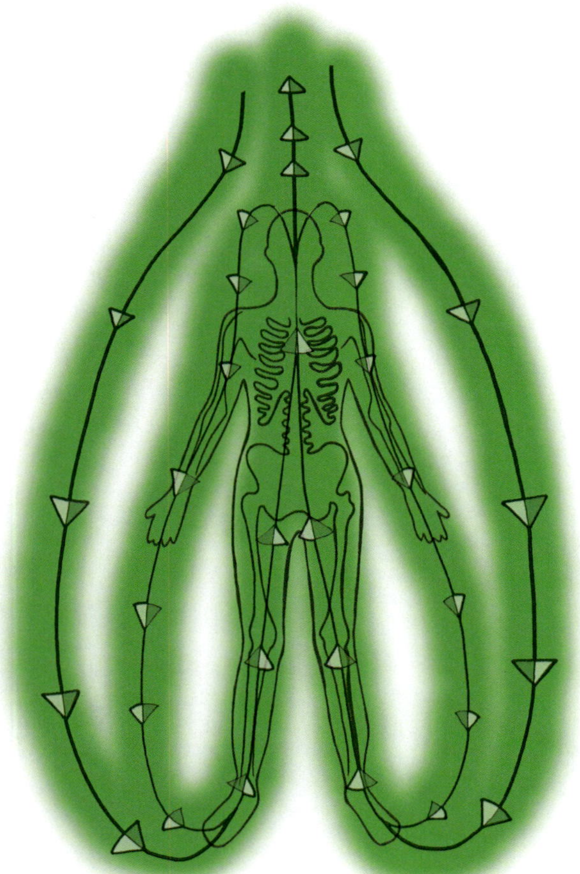

Part VII

Janet's Articles

Family

I love spending time with my family. A family that I never thought I would have, nor consciously knew existed. A family that began over 20 years ago when I first met Stewart and my life was forever changed.

I had a choice. If I had not gone to New York to meet Stewart, I used to wonder what would have happened to me. I think I would have gotten sick and died, or my husband at the time might have killed me. Instead, after I left my then-husband he became very ill, eventually dying a few years after I left. I think because I stopped carrying his load and concentrated on my own. And, perhaps my leaving freed him to move on, too.

Like so many people, I was eager to escape my birth family; to be on my own. Like so many people, I moved away, but I never left the lessons of my birth family behind. Without realizing it, my mind-pattern simply brought my birth family back to me. Different names, different genetics, different locations, but underlying it all, the same people.

My first husband was my mother. Same attributes but in a different body. All my female friends eventually stabbed me in the back—same thing my mom would do. Yet, I never turned my back on my mom. I have worked and worked and worked some more on the issues that I have with her. Because of this, I eventually drew in female friends who supported me. Then, like my mom, I found that those who I thought were my closest friends could only go "so far."

Choices were made and my "friends" removed themselves from my life. It was like a death, losing so many people at once. I cried, I grieved, and finally I let go of the last vestiges of sadness and disappointment.

Interestingly enough, new people who reflect my current self-status filled in the blanks. I re-focused and re-evaluated not only self-expectations but my life-expectations. I think I was so wrapped up in a "set" way of doing things that I closed doors before they could even open to new opportunities.

The fact that people removed themselves from my life tells me that I am completely finished with the mind-patterns that they represented. There was nothing left within my mind-pattern for them to connect. No matching archetypes, colors, or tones. Nada. Nyet. None.

Instead of grieving, I learned to celebrate; to think in new ways and explore new opportunities that suddenly appeared, without second-guessing my Self and with a new sense of confidence, purpose and attitude.

This is where I see you going. But you must, must, must, complete the old first. You cannot move forward until you are willing to face the aspects of your Self that exist within a specific energetic strata. You came here with a purpose. You must complete the foundation before the purpose takes shape. You must ensure the foundation will last and hold up the new house, because most likely there is going to be a "whole lot of shakin' going on."

I continually tell you that your physical structure can only hold "x" amount of experiences. You are here as a finger of the God-Mind so that It can explore Itself. As you know your Self, the God-Mind knows Itself. To completely understand every experience, you must understand both the positive and negative aspects of both. This explains the two sides of the same coin. Only then can you move on.

Your first experiences are your foundational ones. The ones that represent the mind-patterns that allowed you to enter this Physical Reality in the first place. You had to have matching mind-patterns, aka Color, Tone, and Archetype with your birth parents in order to be born; to be drawn from the nonphysical into the physical. This is why you *chose* your parents.

You must understand your own foundation before you can move into something bigger and better. Otherwise your foundation will be weak and it will fall, collapsing all that you have cobbled together. This is one reason why the cycle of birth and death exists. To allow you the opportunity to get the basics down so you can stop repeating them.

Life is not that complicated, instead it is you who complicate life when you run away from it. Run toward your life with all your heart and soul. Embrace what you have and be grateful for the opportunities to stretch beyond your comfort zone.

God knows that I have been stretched further than I would have ever consciously dreamed. But, I have survived, surpassed, become stronger and will continue to grow wiser. There is no limit to what I can do as long as I follow and respect Universal Law. I am thrilled to know that you care enough about your own journey to consider what I have been through, to use my experiences to help you objectively evaluate your own life. This is why I continually ask you to explore your own birth family because this represents your own foundational mind-patterns with which you entered this reality. You cannot escape them because somewhere, somehow, they *are* You!

Family is a Trigger Word

This is one of the biggest trigger words that exist within the language of humanity. This word is the most reactionary word known to humankind. Regardless of color, race, religion, gender, or country, this one word evokes a reaction of some kind from every single living human being. These reactions range from nostalgia to fear to downright hatred. I believe that I have seen every emotion known to humankind when I start bringing up family relationships.

This word is so emotionally-charged that you forget that you chose to be born. You chose where, how, with whom, and when. Your mind-pattern brought you here under your specific circumstances. Why do you not remember? Because you needed to start over with the opportunity to "get it right" this time. You needed to focus on the here and now. Not other lifelines and other possibilities. Focusing in the present is tough. It is a kindness that the distractions are removed for you. You needed to know something up close and personal that will forge your soul-personality in a way that nothing else can.

At the moment of conception, your birth parents opened a pathway for you from the nonphysical into the physical. You had to have matching mind-patterns somewhere to draw you to them. You did not arrive here by chance. There was something specific you needed for balance. The two people you chose as your entry point into this reality were the most perfect fit for you at the time.

Any issues you have with your parents did not start with these two people. These people are only the outpicturing of what was already within you, somewhere, some place. Or, they demonstrate a potential negative (or positive) mind-pattern unless you change.

This is a challenging concept. You may not see this within yourself. Especially if you have been running away from your family or from what your family represents. Some people change their names. Females most often opt out of carrying the family name by taking on her partner's last name. You may go by a nickname or childhood version of your given name. You determinedly lose your chosen name to embrace something new because you are running away from an uncompleted task.

Your first name represents your conscious connection to the outer world. Changing your first name changes the way that you interact with the world. If you shorten your first name, then you shorten the amount of frequency that you allow to flow through you. Look at the letters you choose to eliminate. What aspects of Self do these represent (review the chart in *Healer's Handbook*) that you do not allow yourself to express? If you choose a childhood nickname, then you have a part of you that is stuck in childhood. Totally changing your first name means total denial of your pre-birth agreement deciding how you would interact with the world.

The middle name represents your subconscious mind. You need a middle name as your physical representation of your subconscious mind connection between conscious and superconscious minds. Most importantly, the middle name provides the energetic frequency necessary for left and right brain hemispheres to connect and synchronize. Without this frequency connection your life experiences will have a tendency to go the extreme, both positive and negative. If you have more than one middle name, you open yourself up to alters, subpersonalities, and self-sabotage. "Too many cooks spoil the broth" is an appropriate saying in this case.

The surname represents your superconscious mind. This is your connection to your Oversoul and God-Mind. Your birth surname is the frequency through which you naturally connect Self to Oversoul and God-Mind. If you do not use your last name, you are cutting off your spiritual connection.

Evaluate your life to determine if you have run away from your birth origins in any way. There is a difference between completing your foundations and running away/ignoring them. If your family members are the ones who cut the ties, then this can be a thankful release with the hidden message that you have completed all the lessons that this set of circumstances held for you.

When you cut the ties, then you have to look at the reasons why. I have clients who have cut the ties but instead of growing into something better, have grown into the mind-patterns of those family members they like the least.

This is because the strength of their focus pulls to them exactly what they are trying to avoid. Compare this to something that you read about in the papers very often—auto accidents. There will be one lone tree in some field, or to the side of the road. This is what the driver hits. Why? Because when a vehicle is out of control, the focus is to avoid the tree. The strength of the focus is so strong that the mind-pattern automatically pulls the vehicle into the tree.

"Whatever you hate, you become." Same reasoning with your

family. What you seek to avoid often becomes your focus. Therefore, while you seek to avoid certain behaviors your inherent mind-pattern exists and is genetically as well as subconsciously reinforced.

This is why you see the same health issues repeated in family lineages. The propensity is within you. How latent or active the mind-pattern is depends upon what you do with the raw material. The basic raw material is your Mind.

There is a difference between:

- Ignoring something and pretending it does not exist.
- Running away from something you know does exist.
- Facing the issue, greeting the challenge, and surpassing the mind-pattern so it does not have to be repeated.

You may think you have moved through an issue when you simply are so tightly locked into the first two bullets above that you do not realize what you are doing. Objectivity, as discussed in my *Decoding Your Life* book, is a basic that you need on this journey. Objectivity is something that most people lack.

You must be able to see both the positive and the negative of every situation before you are completely finished. This is the only way to be completely finished with any mind-pattern in this reality.

With all of this in mind, recognize that running away and/or ignoring your birth family is only running away from your Self—something that you can never do.

Family of Choice

Most people have some kind of "family of choice." You may have a life partner, children, in-laws, friends, Internet acquaintances, and even colleagues, co-workers, and/or neighbors who are like family. Literally.

This means that each one of these people represent some aspect of your birth family, either positive or negative; sometimes both. What you do not work out with your birth family you set up and repeat with others in your life. Because of this, every relationship that is honest has both positives and negatives. You came into a reality of duality. You came to explore your positive and negative aspects. If you only see one side of someone, then there is something that you are missing.

People who only show the positive are hiding their negative side. People who show only the negative are hiding their positive side.

When you come across people like this, pay attention. This is an obvious sign that something is not as it appears to be. Everyone is a combination of both positive and negative. Everyone is a microcosm of the macrocosm. Because this is a reality of duality, every person has the potential to express both sides of the spectrum. The ideal is a balance of positive and negative, with *you* being in charge of what you express and when you express, *not* the positive or negative being in charge of *you*.

For example, if someone or something upsets you, you need to go to center to objectively observe what is happening and why. If it is appropriate, then you may need to express some negative aspect to get your point across. You use your emotion; your emotion does not use you.

In the same way, if someone or something pleases you, you need to go to center to objectively observe what is happening and why. If it is appropriate, then you may need to express some positive aspect to get your point across. You use your emotion; your emotion does not use you.

People often understand the negative but are more challenged to understand the positive, so examine this scenario a little closer. Say someone does something wonderful for you. You need to know why—is this person genuine or is this person manipulating you? Is the person controlling you to get something that is more beneficial for him/her than for you? You may get so caught up in the "wonderful" outer appearance that you lose your objectivity over the event.

This happens often in relationships. I hear, "he's so wonderful; she's amazing, etc.," so then I have to add, "Yes, but there are always two sides to every person. What is the other side? Have you seen this yet?"

You can get so caught up in a person, idea, place, or even a thing that your dreams are not based upon reality. Your dreams can be based upon where you want to be, but you have not yet created that foundation upon which your dreams can not only stand, but thrive and develop.

You cannot have the perfect relationship that you dream about when you have not balanced your foundational mind-pattern with the people who first imprinted you in this reality—your birth mother and birth father.

You are always going to be dissatisfied until you correct the deepest layers upon which you base your current life. This is why people continually choose the same person except in a different body. The inherent mind-pattern is the strongest; it is the most suppressed and therefore has gathered the most strength. It lies there, waiting to spring out when you least expect it. Why? Because it is buried and consciously forgotten. When you relax, forgetting to add more dirt so it cannot escape, a little air pocket develops until...whooosh…out it comes! Surprise! Or not…

Because a part of you knows that it exists. You have ignored it or run away from it. Because this is the "easiest" way to get through life. Until one day, you cannot ignore it any longer. It is in front of your face. Then you become upset, depressed, and sometimes inconsolable, wishing for an end to your miserable life.

Once you realize that ultimately, this is only a result of your own mind-pattern, you get real with your Self. You have to. "Wherever you go, there you are." It does not matter where you move, what job change you have, what partners or friends come into your life, if you stay in body or move out of body, everything underlying all is still the same because *you* are still the same.

If this person did not do it "to you" someone else would have. Because *you* are the same. Stop blaming other people, places, or things. Look within. Look without. Deal with your family of choice.

These people provide your closet support system, whether you recognize this or not. You may think of "support system" as a positive and you wonder where they are. However, your support system can also support your negative aspects. When you examine this twist, you may be surprised at the support system you have created for your Self.

Make a list of your current "family of choice," whoever they might be. On your list, determine if the person supports you positively or negatively. And, how. Finally, make a note of who this person represents in your birth family—mother, father, brother, sister.

This helps you recognize what life-patterns you continue to replicate as well as the origins of the mind-pattern that creates the life-pattern.

Family of choice is an outpicturing of your mind-patterns. Family of choice is a replication of your birth family. Family of choice is still all about *you*. Rough stuff, sometimes, but you have to get through it so you can move on and surpass. You have the tools; you are gaining awareness. You can do it. This is your First and Foremost reason for entering this reality—to create a foundation so that you can move forward. I challenge you to not only step up to the task, but to complete it. Do you accept this challenge?

Artificial Family...

The next plan for humanity.

Old term: "Surrogate Mother."
Replacement term: "Gestational Surrogate."

Old term: "Surrogate"
Replacement term: "Carrier."

New Term: "Gestational Carrier."
Next Stop: Artificial Womb.

What happens when you are born in an artificial womb?

Who becomes your initial mind-pattern imprinter?

Who is your family?

Where is your allegiance?

What if you are a clone? and you look around, seeing multiples of your Self looking back at you?

What is the lesson of the soul-personality who makes these choices?

Would you trade your current birth family for the choice to come into this reality via an artificial womb? and/or a clone?

How would your life be different?

Would you be a better person because of it?

Merging Your Family Within

- Lifelines…simultaneous; on-world; off-world; interdimensional.
- Sub-personalities…parts of Self coalesced into consciousnesses that act independent of you.
- Emotions…positive; negative; neutral.
- Alters…artificially programmed; fractured via personal trauma; inner child.
- Cellular intelligence…individual cells; groups of cells; visceral organs; bones; muscles; and so forth.
- Psychic attachments…from you to others, places, and things.
- Astral attachments…out-of-body entities; collective unconscious; demons; dark forces.
- Oversoul…your point of origin out of the God-Mind; your soul-personality's parent
- God-Mind…your Oversoul's point of origin out of the Absolute/All That Is; your Oversoul's parent

Wolf Frequency = Family Frequency

Wolf Frequency is closely associated with clan and family, enhancing the development of close family relationships, good times between people or groups of people, and camaraderie.

Wolf Frequency is warm, caring, and nurturing, with an aggressive side that is only excited and activated during family crises or attacks by others.

Wolf Frequency finds strong support and aid from those around him/her in times of crisis.

Wolf Frequency, when used by couples, creates sexual devotion to one another and enjoyment of life together.

Wolf Frequency helps you to understand hard times and dark energies, as well as to surpass them.

Wolf Frequency enables you to get yourself out of many predicaments and challenging life situations in an efficient manner.

Wolf Frequency makes child-rearing easier.

Wolf Frequency promotes a sense of loyalty and respect, supporting anyone who has been sexually abused, or who has suffered alienation, isolation, and/or abandonment.

Wolf Frequency helps merge and coalesce both your Inner and Outer Family.

Family Affirmations

I make peace with the circumstances of my birth.

I accept and like my self-chosen birth name.

I communicate with all birth family members, both in and out-of-body, via the Oversoul level.

I merge with all aspects of my birth family, both positive and negative.

I make peace with my birth family.

I make peace within my Self.

I surpass the genetic lineage of my birth family.

Family Visualization/Meditation

- Breathe your Self into Your Center with your focus at your pineal gland.
- Breathe out through the top of your head, up to your Oversoul and up into God-Mind.
- With your Mind, will your auric field in close to your body so that you know where it starts and where it stops.
- Surround your auric field with a violet bubble with a mirror on the outside.
- Breathe your Self in and breathe your Self out.
- Visualize your current family, beginning with the person who most influences you now. This can be a positive influence or a negative influence.
- With your Mind, create the Brown Merger Archetype passing through this person.
- Create the same passing through you.
- With your Mind, pull this person into your Brown Merger Archetype until both are Merged.
- Continue this process with each person of your current family.
- Observe how you feel as you do this with each person.
- Understand what the person reflects back to you as you move through your list of family.
- When you are done, release everything back to your Oversoul.
- Repeat this exercise at least once per day for the next 30 days.
- Observe how your feelings change, if any.

I am grateful for my birth family.

Finding Your Voice

Most people think that communication is about exchanging ideas and getting along. This is the truth in True Reality. In the reality of Illusion, in which most people live, most communication has become a free-for-all in which people use information for control of others, almost much like a weapon.

Everyone has lots of conversations going on in their heads all the time. But, how many of these conversations are actually openly communicated to others? Every time you open your mouth, you are subject to ridicule. For this reason, it is easier for most people to close down their ability to communicate, preferring to keep conversations light and casual.

For most people, the shut-down of the communication process starts almost as soon as you begin to communicate. There is a difference between parental direction of proper, socially-accepted methods of communication, and parental behavior leading to total shut-down. As a child, it is important to learn when to speak and when not to speak, how to wait your turn before speaking, acceptable voice levels, speaking instead of crying, etc. These are necessary social behaviors that everyone needs to master.

However, often children's thoughts and opinions are not valued and considered by the adults in their lives. Sometimes children's opinions are laughed at or ridiculed. This soon teaches the child to keep his/her thoughts to him/herself. Perhaps every time the child speaks, someone interrupts, never letting the child finish. Perhaps an honest opinion from a child is seen as rude or impudent, and the child is punished. If you think about it, you probably have some communication story from your childhood that left a lasting impression.

The same thing happens to adults. They merely repeat with each other what they learned from their parents as children, or perhaps in school, or from other adult role models. One moment you share an intimate thought with someone that you trust. The next minute the person turns against you, using your own words against you like a weapon. This double-strike is exceptionally painful. These experiences stay with you.

Each communication try that ends in emotional or physical wounding stays with you. Eventually, communication skills deteriorate. It becomes increasingly difficult to let anyone know what you think or how you feel. You are lucky if you have a person or two with whom you can share your deepest thoughts, but even this poses a risk. If you have communication difficulties with these close people, which is normal, then the pain can become even deeper.

Mind-patterns develop that say you are not worthy of being heard, that your opinions are not important, and that vocalizations are emotionally and physically painful. These all feed into victim-mentality and low self-worth issues.

Once you realize this, then it is important that you release your old ideas of communication so that you can begin building new mind-patterns that allow you to express who and what you are. Social manners and responsibilities are always important. This means you must still be conscious of when you speak and how you speak, but as you develop and improve upon your communication skills, victim-mentality recedes and self-worth improves.

The beginning step is just learning to open your mouth. This is easy enough to implement by getting some practice in speaking out loud—even be to yourself! The important thing is to find your voice and exercise it, just as you would exercise any muscle that is weak from lack of use.

Toning is a great way to find your voice. Go into your shower with the water running and simply allow yourself to make some noise. Or, stand by the edge of a large body of water, such as lake or ocean, and make noise with your voice. Exercise your vocal cords so they know what it is like to let loose all the suppressed tones, noises, and words that have been pushed into them for years, perhaps even lifelines.

As the sounds come forth, mentally start allowing shapes, colors, and images to pass before your mental eye. Take some time to explore anything that is particularly interesting for any reason, either positive or negative, or maybe even just intriguing.

Spend time with yourself, expressing and releasing from the vocal cords as much as you can of all that has been suppressed within them.

As you exercise them, you will notice that they become more supple and your vocal range extends. This allows you to explore further suppressions as well as opens you to the communication process in new and interesting ways.

This newfound strength of vocal communication soon extends to the outer world. You will find yourself speaking up more and more. You will realize that suppressed communication was "natural" to you due to the mind-pattern imprinting. Now, with your practiced vocal freedom, you will find that you naturally express your thoughts, feelings, and opinions. Knowing that your thoughts and opinions are worth stating, you will find that you react less to the reactions of others. You become more balanced and centered, and self-worth and self-identity increases.

Finding your voice means liberating your vocal cords. These are the tools through which you communicate your words. You are cleaning them up so that they can do what they came here to do. You allow them to express the words that you wanted to speak or say for years and year, and even eons of time.

Finding your voice also means better physical health. Sore throats are about repressed expressions. Any illness of the throat, including thyroid issues, has to do with speaking up for yourself. Look at the mind-patterns behind the body part, and you will know exactly what suppressed and repressed mental state brought the physical body to a state of negative health.

Finding your voice means finding an open flow of communication, where you can build your bridges with the outer world in a way where you become increasingly comfortable with your own thoughts, opinions, and feelings. The more comfortable you are with your own expressions, the greater the flow of outer communication. Unleashing the power of your voice unleashes incredible personal power in astonishing ways! Go for it!

God-Mind Logic

Most people think in terms of linear logic because this is the way they are trained. Linear logic means that if you do "x" then "y" will follow. For example, if you study hard in school (x) then you will get good grades (y). Or, if you put a pot of water on a hot burner (x) then the water will eventually boil. The world is full of such neat and precise logical situations, always moving you from Point A to Point B to Point C and so forth, in a straight "linear" line.

There are numerous books designed to teach you how to think using linear logic. The entire educational system enforces linear logic. The more education you have the more linear logic is expected of you. After all, how can you function unless you can project what effect "x" will have on "y"?

Studying linear logic (x) affects *you* by narrowing your focus away from multidimensional logic (y)—another brilliant and well-implemented plan to keep you away from the capabilities of your true self. Because you are so accustomed to thinking linearly, thinking in multidimensional logic, which is your natural state, becomes a challenge.

Always remember that you are a microcosm of the macrocosm, and as such, whatever is within God-Mind is within you. God-Mind does not "think" in linear terms. This is why events in your life appear to happen haphazardly. From a linear logical standpoint, there is no order, only chaos.

To truly understand the scenario of life, one must move into the True Nature of True Reality, which does not run in a straight line from Point A to Point B to Point C. This is why you can plan and plan, and plan some more, yet what you think is going to happen never happens, or happens in a completely different way than you ever imagined. This is because you live in a linear box.

True geniuses always think "outside the box"—the linear box, that is. True geniuses do not let the constraints of the educational system box them in. They constantly daydream and allow their minds to wander into the world of "what if" without limitations. They get off the linear line. True greats are often described as "they did it their own way" or "they had their own style" or even, "they were completely self-taught."

When you put your requests out to your Oversoul and God-Mind, sometimes it appears that your requests are denied or not even heard. This is because once you do this, you create a picture in your own mind of how and when your request will be answered. In True Reality, as soon as you make the request there is an answer, but most of the time you do not recognize it.

If you request a beautiful new car but do not know how to drive, manifesting one immediately might not be the most appropriate action for you at the moment. Maybe your personality is rash and would not properly handle the responsibility of piloting a mass of steel down the highway. Maybe your personality would need some adjustments before you could even deal with a driving instructor. Maybe your area does not have proper roads. Or, maybe the roads you have will soon be under construction, but you do not know this yet.

Maybe if you have a car too soon, someone might get hurt. Maybe "your car" is not ready for you yet—the correct frequency of your vehicle is extremely important since your car is an outpicturing of you. This list of "maybes" can go on and on, and maybe all of the above describes you! So, before the car manifests, you have a lot to get in order.

Yet, the impatient you might not recognize the maybes. You might think "I want one *now*" and "No one is listening." Maybe someone *is* listening, but sees the dangers in immediate manifestation and prefers to get you in order first so that when the time comes you can handle the responsibility and all that comes with owning a car.

So, instead of driving your beautiful sleek car that you envision, life becomes more challenging and complicated. Unbeknownst to you, these are the challenges that make you ready for the correct car at the correct time. You become frustrated that nothing is happening and your mood swings run from ranting and raving to feeling sorry for yourself.

All the while, your Oversoul and God-Mind are doing everything in their power to get you to the point where you can have your car. But because you did not recognize these steps to getting there, you feel let down and denied. The linear logic of your mind already sets up the path of how and when your car is arriving. Since this is not happening, obviously something is wrong—with you, the system, your Oversoul/God-Mind connections, etc. Frustration builds and eventually you give up.

Once you give up and stop trying to direct the action, your Oversoul and God-Mind can work more quickly and efficiently. You may still see the challenges as overwhelming and defeating. You may choose to beat yourself up, or you may greet the challenges as you conclude that you have no choice anyway.

God-Mind is much too vast for anyone to grasp Its workings in Its entirety, yet people often feel frustrated with themselves for not understanding. Why is that? Accept the fact that God-Mind has an entirely different set of logic than the system in which you are trained.

Release your linear logic, and embrace your True Nature of multidimensional God-Mind logic. Understand that you may *not* always understand the why's and how's of your life until the event is complete and you are able to look back, study, and release. This is how you remember and re-embrace your multidimensional self—through experiential learning. How can one really teach you about something that you must experience?

If you have closed yourself off to your True Nature, then your True Nature must be re-opened, and re-learned, or re-membered so that you can get back into the True Nature of Self. You can learn to look, plan, and dream beyond linear logic. You can visualize "wild and crazy" scenarios without limitations and then allow them to happen rather than squeeze them out by trying to force a linear, logical series of events your way.

Remember, you can force your way, but that does not mean this brings the best results. By doing so you squeeze out what your Oversoul and God-Mind have planned for you. Your proactive participation in your multidimensional self allows for the macrocosm to become more fully functional in Its way once again. Why set your life up so that It must fight you to give you what you want? How crazy of a system is this that you have studied and accepted?

God-Mind Logic is definitely *not* linear logic; God-Mind *contains* linear logic, but also contains a multitude of other kinds of logic that are an important part of the functioning of all realities—including your current one!

Group Consciousness vs. Individualized Consciousness

The work that I do has provided me with an interesting journey, to say the least. One of the most challenging aspects is explaining to people what I do. Everyone wants to fit me into a specific category, into some kind of "group" so that they can begin to understand. They want to be able to relate me to something.

There does not seem to be a neat package to explain my work. I have not found a group with a simple description that I can share with others. Those who have a group tend to alienate me. If you do not understand something, or someone, then get rid of them!

I learned long ago not to expect anything from anyone. Then I would not be disappointed. If, by chance, I received something positive, I was pleasantly surprised. I decided I would rather have the occasional reward versus the continual disappointments. This took me many years to understand why.

I found my answer when I started exploring the concept of the Group Consciousness vs. Individualized Consciousness.

I realized at the time that everything has a Consciousness. When you are a child in school, you are taught about "animate" vs. "inanimate" objects. Yet, my research even as a young child showed me that absolutely everything in existence has a Consciousness.

I learned to tap into the Consciousness of everything around me, whether it was a rock, tree, insect, Earth, sky, or a cell within my body. I found Consciousness everywhere. If you are entrained in conventional education, you have to open yourself to explore this concept. Otherwise, you are going to be stuck in the "alive" vs "not alive" mentality.

Realize that even as an "outside of the box thinker" you still operate within specific parameters that need to be broken through. In my book, *Decoding Your Life,* I explain that you have to find new questions so you can get new answers so you can ask new questions again. Vertical growth is a process that my entire body of work advocates and encompasses.

I never saw my Self as part of the Group consciousness. I was outside of this energy mass. I am Individualized Consciousness. I am a drop of water within the ocean, but I am not the ocean. I am the drop of water that has made its way into a bay, into a river, then a stream, and now just one tiny drop. Yet, the same components within that drop are also within the ocean. One individualized drop of water.

Moving out of Group Consciousness into Individualized Consciousness is a challenge. I am sure you know this from the experiences within your own life. What you may not realize is that this is a natural process that sooner or later, all aspects of the God-Mind go through.

This is why there is such a struggle as you move into this phase of your existence. You actually move through the mass of Group Consciousness, pushing farther and farther away from it. The suction of the Group Consciousness pull is enormous as you go through the extrication process.

Group Consciousness is answering the question for the God-Mind, "What is Group Consciousness?" You are a part of the answer. Your participation as well as your extrication from it defines this aspect of the God-Mind.

This is why the more that you think for your Self (Individualized Consciousness) the harder the Group Consciousness works to pull you back in. Because if each cell within Group Consciousness transcends the Group, the Group Consciousness ceases to exist. When

God-Mind knows what Group Consciousness is, then all the questions will have been asked as well as answered.

You are in the process of transmuting Group Consciousness into something else. The first step is always awareness. The second step is action. Now you are in the process of extricating your Self from one aspect of God-Mind into Something Else.

You are what I call a "Way Show-er." You are forging the path. You are brave. You are strong. There are others, many others, going through this same process of transmutation. You are finding others of like-mind. Re-positioning your Self for your next phase.

Welcome to the World of God-Mind/Oversoul Growth!

Understanding Group Consciousness

Everything in existence comes out of the God-Mind. Therefore, everything is a microcosm of the macrocosm of some part of the God-Mind. You can extrapolate this to mean that if it exists, it has a Consciousness.

Similar Consciousness' gather together. This can be a forest of trees or sand in a desert or rocks in a mountain or cells in a mammal. Consciousness exists beyond any physical object, a large vaporous energy cloud hanging in the air. If you look at these bodies of consciousness, you see the energetic tendrils attached to each outward physical representation.

For example, each tree in the forest appears to be alone, but when you look above the forest, you see the vaporous energy cloud hovering above, with a tendril into each tree. This is how messages get passed through the forest. One tree feels something and passes it through the Group Consciousness on to the next and the next and so forth until all the trees have the same message. Humanity as a whole has a Group Consciousness. There is this same vaporous energy cloud that hangs over humanity. This makes each person look kind of like a puppet on a string. Most people are more outside of the body than in the body. This is why some extremely primitive and aggressive behaviors exist.

These are to make you aware that you even have a body. Pain and discomfort focus your attention to the fact that you have a physical body. Hunger tells you what a stomach is. Torture, beatings, and deprivation force you to focus in this physical reality.

If you want to move into Individualized Consciousness, the first step is to be acutely aware that you have a body; that you exist in this reality; and that there is more to life than the behavior of the group.

Always keep the awareness that God-Mind is "All One." Remove one "L." "L" is the Hyperspace Archetype for "homebody." Removing this archetype releases you from your metaphorical home. You are now free to venture out on your own—"A lone." You have removed your Self from the Group Consciousness of "All One" into Individualized Consciousness of "A Lone."

Group Consciousness is reinforced in the womb, when your consciousness is intertwined with that of your mother's. Upon birth, you are intertwined with your birth father, siblings, and other relatives. All these people are intertwined with you, whether this entwinement is positive or negative. You are part of a Group Consciousness whether it is functional or dysfunctional. When your group is together, you feel whole and complete. This is a reminder of the Group Consciousness of your Origins; of the God-Mind Itself. When your Group Consciousness is physically separated, you feel alone and frustrated.

As a child, you are not aware of the difference between Group and Individual. Everyone is one and the same. You assume that everyone is the same as you, wanting the same things at the same time. You have no boundaries, borders, or individual identity. You have no concept of "yours and mine." As far as you are concerned "what's yours is mine and what's mine is mine."

You do not realize the boundaries that exist until you are taught that there are boundaries. You may have been demonstrative, hugging and kissing everyone. You assume everyone wants to be hugged and kissed until you are told that this is not so...and in fact, in some circumstances not appropriate at all.

You sing and laugh loudly; cry and scream when you are in emotional pain; talk in public like you are the only person in existence. You have to be taught that there are other people and must be respectful of their space. You have no idea that others may perceive your actions as an annoyance or irritation because you are still in Group Consciousness Mode.

Group Consciousness is a strong part of self-survival. You may not know why, but you know you need your original Group Consciousness—your family. When they do not come through for you, you spend your entire life trying to recreate the same group in bits and pieces so that you can bring those parts of Self back together—to re-integrate and merge all aspects of your Group Consciousness together.

Of course, you recognize now that the outer world is merely a reflection of your own inner world. By re-integrating the bits and pieces of your Self, the rest of your world comes together.

This is the continual process—understanding your own Individualized Consciousness in its entirety so that you can unite with other similar ones. But, while maintaining your own individualized Self is now extremely important, there is always the pull to re-unite with the God-Mind Itself.

Your soul-personality is now on its journey into Individualized Consciousness. "A lone." But most importantly, you are no longer "A lone" as we join together on our journey into Individualized Consciousness. In this step, we are like a giant battery. Together, we retain our individuality while boosting each other to new heights in this continual exploration of the God-Mind. You are "A lone" in a new way. Respectful of borders and boundaries, aware that others exist with unique needs and requirements, but honoring the entire process.

Everyone and everything will eventually go through this same journey. Out of the Group Conscious into Individualized Consciousness. For this reason, it is important for you to not only understand what you are going through, but have compassion for your own process. Others have gone before you; others will follow. Explore as you go, always sending your findings up to your Oversoul and back to the God-Mind, your Source and Point of Origin.

Artificially Created Group Consciousness aka Mind-Control

Group Consciousness is easier to control than Individualized Consciousness. There are many societal groups formed for the specific reason of Mind-Control. This is to the advantage for anyone wanting to control people. Keep them as one Group Consciousness or, one Mind-Pattern.

- Military
- Prison
- Schools
- Churches
- Government
- Healthcare
- Industry

These are often maintained by:

- Wearing uniforms
- Eating the same food
- Speaking the same words and phrases together
- Keeping the same hours
- Performing the same tasks at the same time
- Reading the same books
- Watching the same television and radio programs
- Exercising together
- Repetition, repetition, repetition.

One Mind-Pattern is easier to control than many separate ones. Observe how Group Consciousness' are artificially created and maintained. Be able to work within it if necessary, but know that you are on your way to Individualized Consciousness.

Individualized Consciousness Means…

I think for myself.

I consider the opinions of others, but am not swayed by them.

Numbers of people thinking one way does not mean I automatically believe that they are correct in their thinking.

I do not jump on board the latest trends.

I am able to balance emotion with logic and logic with emotion.

I remain steadfast in the face of adversity.

I am true to my Self.

I have compassion for the trials of others, but I do not take them on.

I do not allow others to hold me back.

I do not try to drag others with me.

I am willing to try new things "A lone."

I look to my Oversoul and God-Mind for support, even when I may not understand everything I want to understand at the moment.

I trust the process.

I believe in who and what I am.

I can live with my Self at the end of each day.

I am whole and complete exactly as I am.

Mind-Control via Creation of Artificial Group Consciousness

Those who work to control the Global population understand the energetics of Group Consciousness. You need to understand this, too, so you have awareness of what is happening not only to the world around you, but to you, personally, as a result.

Group Consciousness is always in balance. Group Consciousness is equivalent to a moving, breathing entity. Visualize one giant soul-personality expressing through many physical beings of the same kind.

Butterflies, for example, have approximately 30,000 different species expressing through the Butterfly Group Consciousness. Still, each species is unique and each individual within each species is unique. No two butterflies are the same.

All animals are connected to their Oversoul via a Group Consciousness. This is why animals travel in groups. They think as one. They act as one. Each animal knows his/her specific place in the hierarchy; each one knows his/her task. Each animal is a part of the whole, connecting to the emotion/feeling/knowing of the Group Consciousness.

Each animal Group Consciousness is an outer representation of the Human Being Group Consciousness. Those who use mind-control on an unsuspecting population know this. This is why there are conscious efforts to remove or greatly reduce specific animal populations. These specific animal populations hold and anchor specific frequencies from the nonphysical into the physical. When the frequency is no longer strongly represented in this reality, whatever is represented/outpictured by that animal population is forced further inside the Human population.

For example, wolf represents family. Take the Wolf Frequency out of physical reality to represent the break-up of the family. Any animal that is extinct means that that mind-pattern no longer expresses on Earth. Or, more accurately, the specific frequency is suppressed.

Any animal on the "endangered" list represents the diminishment of that quality within the context of the Human Group Consciousness. The Human Group Consciousness cannot express this as easily because it is now suppressed. The doorway between the nonphysical to the physical is either closed, almost closed, or closing.

There are laws that specifically forbid you from eating specific wild game and some that forbid the selling of wild game. This is not simply denying you a specific food—you are literally being denied a specific frequency from the God-Mind. In the United Kingdom it is illegal for anyone to eat "swan" except royalty—specifically, the Queen.

When you ingest a specific food, you actually partake of that frequency. You activate it within yourself. People who eat beef, a domesticated animal, are more likely to have a herd mentality than people who eat buffalo, which is an aggressive animal and harder to contain. One way the white settlers controlled the Group Consciousness of the indigenous people was to eliminate their food source, almost to extinction.

Those who control the food source control the population. What you ingest physically anchors the nonphysical into your body, allowing it to express in and through you. This explains the true meaning of the expression, "you are what you eat."

Animals are put on the endangered list so that you cannot have the frequency within your personal environment; so that you cannot "use" that specific frequency. There is a reason why they are endangered and you are not allowed to eat or own any part of them. There is a faction that allows them to be hunted to extinction for control of the Human Group Consciousness.

Everything "real" is becoming extinct because this prevents specific Group Consciousness' from expressing in this reality. Less outer representation and anchoring of your inner possibilities. More control over you. This is always done so that one Human turns against another. Consider the campaign against wearing real fur. Your emotions are targeted so that you think of the "poor animals," but those behind the movement are cold and calculating. They are only concerned with removing pure animal frequency from your life.

This is why the indigenous peoples dressed in the specific furs, used specific animal parts and ate the flesh of whatever animals they wanted to communicate with. They used tones and dances, which are really a combination of labyrinths and archetypes as their entry code into the frequency.

Indigenous peoples all over the world ate specific animal organs/ body parts to ingest the frequency, or attribute, of that animal. They ate the beating heart of a freshly killed lion, for example, and then utilized every single part of the lion to anchor Lion Frequency. This is why the ways of the indigenous peoples have all been ridiculed and eliminated as "old-fashioned" and "superstition."

The global population was hoodwinked into believing these ancient practices were curiosities to be laughed at while those that formulated these plans stole the knowledge of these peoples and then brought these people to either extinction or the edge of extinction.

Group Consciousness is emotional and is in tune with the feeling nature of whatever species is expressing through it. This is why non-industrialized countries are more about family than industrialized countries. "Non-industrialized" simply means those populations are not as mind-controlled as industrialized populations. Non-industrialized are not developed/mind-controlled...yet. Those who would control the global population are taking over the world one population group at a time. Either control them or eliminate them. Slowly but surely the net is being closed in.

The target is always the Group Consciousness and how to disband/de-energize/prevent its expression here on Earth. Suppress the expression of the Group Consciousness of any species and suppress its expression within the Human population. Force the Human population into one mind-pattern for easier control purposes.

You see this with the elimination not only of animal populations, but also plants and minerals. At one time currency was all minerals—copper, silver, gold, representing strength, Oversoul, and God-Mind. These frequencies are slowly being withdrawn from the population. Someday it may be illegal to own these minerals.

Everything real is being eliminated/suppressed and replaced with artificial. Artificial wood; artificial fabrics; artificial animal artifacts; artificial fabrics; artificial food. The Artificial Group Consciousness is being created and anchored here in this reality. The ultimate goal: Artificial Intelligence, i.e., Mind-Control.

This is why Individualized Consciousness is a threat. If you hang onto any True Frequency you anchor it into physical reality. This keeps something alive and present that is being hunted for complete destruction. This also explains why philosophers, teachers, artists, spiritual leaders, and older people are always targeted for elimination in any takeover. Remove those who anchor specific "undesirable" Group Consciousness,' as well as those who forge the path for the undesired "Individualized Consciousness."

Then, those most susceptible to anchor in the Artificial Intelligence Group Consciousness become the police for those who are not susceptible. Use numbers of people to try to overcome those with Individualized Consciousness, known as "peer pressure." Push these people to do the dirty work. Human against Human. Sit back and watch the results. Mind-control the weakest links to break the entire chain.

Artificial Group Consciousness is well underway. It gathers strength every second of every day. This is why your journey into Individualized Consciousness can sometimes feel overwhelming. This explains why "friend attacks friend." These attacks and efforts to bring you into the fold are relentless. They most likely will not stop until one day you will be so strong that you no longer react to this pursuit. You will surpass and move on into something better that you have only just now begun to imagine. Individualized Consciousness. A new aspect of the journey into the God-Mind.

Individualized Consciousness Affirmations

I recognize Group Consciousness around me.

I release the pull of the Group Consciousness.

I release those who remain behind in the Group Consciousness, allowing them to grow at their pace, not mine.

I release the need to judge and criticize those still entrapped within Group Consciousness.

I move through Group Consciousness into Individualized Consciousness.

I attract others who are moving into Individualized Consciousness.

My movement into Individualized Consciousness is supported on all levels of existence.

Individualized Consciousness Visualization

- I move freely and easily beyond the boundaries of Group Consciousness for I am whole and complete, Individualized Consciousness.
- Self-contained.
- I already have everything within that I need.
- I look around me to find others in similar positions. Leaving the Group Consciousness. Embracing Individualized Consciousness.
- Together we make a stand for Self, whole and complete.
- Each a unique cell within the God-Mind.
- Self-contained.
- With total acceptance for each other as Individualized Consciousness.
- Allowing Personal Power connected to Oversoul Power connected to God-Mind Power to flow freely through me.
- Needing only Me to complete Me.
- Drawing other aspects of the God-Mind who support Individualized Consciousness.
- Like attracts like.
- Supportive. Uplifting. Surpassing. Boosting into the next phase of Humanity.
- Life without struggle. Growth without pain. Whole and Complete.

I am Individualized Consciousness.

Happiness

The search for "happiness" seems to be the pervading theme underlying everything that almost everyone does. How many times have you said or thought, "I could be happy 'if'…" Or, "I will be happy 'when'…"

How many ways have you filled in the rest of the sentence? "I could be happy if/I will be happy when...I have a new car, a different job, my boss retires, my relationship changes, I lose weight, make more money, etc." How many ways and times have you completed these types of sentences?

How many times have you achieved one of the above? Were you happy for a while, and then you started thinking about the next way in which you could fill in the sentence?

At some point in time, you may finally realize that happiness is an elusive term. You may have the feeling of happiness from time to time from outside input, but to sustain that emotion "forever" most likely is not going to happen.

For one thing, happiness must be fulfilled from whatever exists inside of yourself, rather than from an outside source. Trying to fill yourself with happiness from an outside source is the equivalent of trying to fulfill your emotional needs by eating chocolate cake. They both give you an immediate sense of fulfillment, but eventually the moment is going to pass.

This is what forces you to continue your search. When you get that new car, you think of something else that will make you even happier. Or, maybe the payments create distress, or it has mechanical issues, or you wish that you had purchased a different make, model, color, accessories, etc. The circle starts over again. As long as you try to fulfill your emotional requirements from *any* outside source, you will eventually become disillusioned, be it person, place, or thing.

Happiness is a relative term. When you look around, you "should" be able to state numerous reasons why you should be happy, but are you? Think of what other people do not have compared to yourself. Maybe you do not care for your job, but at least you have one. Somewhere, there is some person out there wishing for a job. Regardless of how menial or thankless you consider your position, someone, somewhere, would be happy for the opportunity to be in your place.

Many people place their elusive search for happiness on attaining a specific goal, or "dream." Do you think that once you attain your dream you will be happy? How long have you had your dream? Have you allowed your dream to change with you, or has your dream remained a constant?

Happiness is only one emotion within the circle of life. There are a variety of emotions that comprise your totality. Happiness is only one small part. If you focus on only one part, even when it is developed inside of yourself, it will be out of balance with your other emotional parts.

For example, if fear is not in balance, you may "fear" that you will lose your happiness. If "anger" is not in balance your temper may destroy your happiness. Everything must be in proper alignment for the totality of you to exist in any kind or harmony.

Happiness is an elusive term for most people because they do not have a clue about maintaining the whole person. Happiness by itself and as generally defined in the linear world is never going to happen.

Recognize that happiness is simply part of the whole. Learn to enjoy the richness of every experience, cultivating all parts of self in such a manner that your totality is fulfilled in a deep and satisfying way.

Appreciate every experience for the wealth of knowledge that each one holds, both positive and negative. You will soon realize that the dream of what you once sought was only an illusion. Now, you can replace your old dream of finding happiness with a new dream that evolves in the same way as you

Happiness Archetype is Made of 1 + 1 + 1

Magnificent numbers that signify New Beginnings. Three 1s.

One Body, One Mind, One Soul.

Conscious, superconscious, subconscious.

Past, present, future.

Left brain, pineal gland, right brain.

Triangle. Three sides.

In Hyperspace Language: Perfection.

Dot. In Hyperspace Language: Consciousness.

Medium green. In Hyperspace Language: Emotional Balance.

Put these three together and you have:

HAPPINESS

Laughter Therapy

How much laughter do you have in your life? What makes you go beyond an appreciative chuckle? What pulls out a deep belly laugh—the kind that makes tears roll down your cheeks? What funny moments in your life make you laugh?

Laughter provides an important function for your mental health, which in turn reflects in your physical health.

Laughter:

- Reduces the levels of cortisol—which is a hormone produced by your body when exposed to high levels of stress.
- Lowers blood pressure.

- Increases and improves blood flow—causes endothelium (inner lining of blood vessels) to expand.
- Promotes heart health—due to improved blood flow.
- Boosts your immune system—enables you to fight off illness and recover from sickness more quickly.
- Releases endorphins—these can act like natural pain killers.

One of my favorite jokes, or maybe the only one I know, always makes me laugh:

The elephant said to the man, "How do you breathe through that thing?"

One of my favorite stories:

Stewart was in Singapore, attending an en extremely prestigious concert by well-known violinist. When everything was most quiet, there was a loud explosion that thundered through the concert hall. When he turned to find the source, he realized that the flash in his disposable camera had exploded in his pocket and he had smoke pouring out of his pants! Needless to say, the violinist wasn't the only one the audience was watching! (No, he doesn't know I included this story…you won't tell him, will you?)

I hope you have smiled, chuckled, or even laughed when reading through this—if so, consider your mental, emotional, and physical health uplifted and improved! *This statement not evaluated by the FDA!*

Nor is this one:

Happiness is the antithesis to all ailments.

Happiness Affirmations

I forgive all who I feel took away my happiness.

I let go of my emotional blocks to happiness.

I release my jealousies of others whom I perceive have happiness.

I deserve happiness.

Every cell of my body soaks up the Happiness Frequency.

Happiness tones reverberate throughout every level of my Being.

Happiness floods my soul.

Oversoul Happiness Infusion Visualization

- Breathe yourself into your center.
- Out through the top of your head with your breath; up into your Oversoul and God-Mind.
- Breathe in; breathe out, anchoring yourself in the strength of your Oversoul and God-Mind.
- With your eyes closed, take a look at your auric field. Notice how far it extends from your body.
- With your eyes closed, use your mind to will your auric field in close to your body.
- Surround your auric field with a violet bubble. Now you have boundaries of where you start and where you stop.
- With your mind, will up to your Oversoul all that you no longer need.
- Mentally create a medium green three-sided pyramid within the bubble that contains you.
- Visualize yourself at the center of this medium three-sided pyramid.
- Notice that the pyramid is flooded with the color of medium green.
- Allow the medium green to flood every cell of your being.
- Breathe in medium green. Observe the medium green pushing out all that you no longer need.
- Exchange what you no longer need for medium green. Infuse every cell of your being on every level with medium green.

- Feel yourself emotionally whole, well, and complete. Allow Happiness to infuse every cell.
- Steep all parts of your Being in Happiness.
- Know Happiness, Breathe Happiness, Be Happiness.
- Breathe Happiness in, Breathe Happiness out.
- Remember the feeling so that you can touch into it wherever you are.

Happiness is Yours for the Taking.

11 Secrets to Sustain Happiness

1. Release your old baggage. "Ignoring" does not mean "released."
2. Release your need to judge and criticize yourself.
3. Make attainable goals that set you up for success.
4. Acknowledge every accomplishment as "success" to imprint this mind-pattern.
5. Focus on what you have accomplished rather than what you have not.
6. Interpret "failure" as "re-direction."
7. Persevere.
8. Turn your lemons into lemonade.
9. Redefine your goals as necessary.
10. Be kind, compassionate, and understanding with yourself.
11. Keep Self, Oversoul, and God-Mind in alignment.

I am One with Happiness.

Introvert, Extrovert

I could never describe myself as an Extrovert. As a child I loved being the center of attention, but I was unable to speak up for myself. I found ways to make myself noticeable such as good grades, doing what others' wanted, and behaving. I thought being noticed meant being "loved."

I had one college professor that said I could not think for myself and only copied the ideas of others. I was mortified. I was in business for myself at the time. I always considered myself highly creative and focused. While I still had an issue with speaking up, I tearfully made my way to the department head to explain my side of the story. She determined that the professor had issues and was taking it out on me.

As I internalized during this time period, my body shut down. I developed perpetual diarrhea during the school quarter. In addition, I developed severe allergies, skin rashes, menstrual issues and asthma, which eventually turned into walking pneumonia. The more I internalized, the more my body outpictured this. The negative energy that I felt was destroying my body.

My vision started shutting down when I was about eight years old. My teeth were crooked as my ability to adjust was sorely lacking. I had numerous earaches because I did not want to hear what was being said. I was shutting all my body systems down. I could not relate to the outer world. I was miserable inside and out.

As a child, I thought the other children would grow into responsible adults. What I learned was that wild children grow into wild adults. The child within never grows up because all energy is pushed inward.

My hobbies were reading, reading, and more reading. Internal escape. More introversion. I loved to write and be by myself because with myself I was never misunderstood. I could do what I wanted without judgment or criticism.

When I wrote my first book in my mid-twenties, I thought the "hard" part was done. I learned that writing the book was the easy part; selling it was another story. Speaking in front of audiences used to make me go weak in the knees and my mind go blank. I could not even focus on my notes.

Eventually I learned that when I took the emphasis off "me" and onto "what do others need," I reached another level of information delivery. I was told via my Oversoul that because no one else was doing what I was doing, it was my "job" to put this information out. Otherwise, who else would do it?

This bit of knowledge changed my perspective, motivating me to speak up. As my ability to speak in public grew, so did my ability to speak in all areas of my life. I no longer withheld my thoughts, but openly expressed what I thought, when I thought. I had to learn balance. I had to listen to my Oversoul for direction. Another tough lesson with sometimes tough consequences. Introvert, extrovert. Finding the Balance. An important aspect of Self-Development.

By Nature, I am an introvert. By conscious design, I am an Extrovert. Combine these together and you have what I AM.

Take a look at your own personal tendencies. Are you an Introvert who needs to bring in some Extrovert qualities to your life? Or, are you an Extrovert who needs to add some Introvert qualities to your personal recipe?

In this reality of duality, Balance is the Key, moving toward Neutrality. This is the point where the evolutionary process of your Soul moves into a new upward evolutionary spiral.

I am a Balance of Introvert and Extrovert Qualities.

Are You an Introvert?

- Did you close down the "real you" many years ago without realizing what you were doing?
- Did/do you hold silent conversations in your head that never left your mouth?
- Did/do you have opinions that you knew no one would appreciate?
- Do you want to please people but are not sure how?
- Are you highly observant?
- Do you feel underestimated?
- Do you have pent-up emotions?
- Do you have vision issues, specifically not being able to see clearly in the distance?
- Are you overweight because this is one way you cannot be overlooked even with a closed mouth?
- Do you have thyroid issues from not speaking up?
- Do you have tongue irregularities from "biting or holding your tongue"?
    - Jaw issues from "biting the bullet" and/or not opening your mouth and/or moving ahead despite your misgivings?
    - Ear problems from not wanting to hear the world around you?
    - Malfunctioning heart and failing internal organs from pulling your psychic energy inward to the point of extinction?
    - Blood issues for not letting joy into your life?
    - Body cramps because you do not want to move into your life?

- Did you feel "safe" in your own home?
- Do you feel like the "real you" is trapped inside and you cannot share this part of yourself with anyone?
- Do you stay in your home rather than mingle with others, often refusing opportunities to socialize?
- When you are with others, do you find it difficult to speak, so you do other things to get attention, from standing on the sidelines to making your presence known in nonverbal ways?
- Did you speak up in another lifeline and get punished for it?
- Were you an inappropriate extrovert that was suddenly reprimanded?
- Did you stand up for something righteous yet evil prevailed?
- Did your words cause you punishment, pain, and /or torture?
- What is your genetic heritage? Were "your people" punished and tortured?
- Were you of the ruling class where your servants did everything for you and now, without your servants you do not know what to do or say?
- Are your internal organs "stopped up" and clogged?
- Do you have a digestive system that does not absorb properly?

The number one fear of most people is public speaking. Speaking in front of others. Yes, you have great conversations in your head, but why can you not let others know what you think? Do your knees quiver and go limp? Does your heart palpitate, thudding in your ears? Does your mind suddenly go blank the minute you make a move to open your mouth? Why?

What is the origin of your inability to speak up for yourself? For most people, this begins with parents who for one reason or another do not let you be who you are as a child. Or, from religious institutions, school, doctors, and others who tried to control, manipulate, and berate you.

Were you allowed to have an opinion? If you stated your opinion, were you punished for it? Did anyone make fun of and ridicule you?

However, for this to happen, you have to come in with the propensity to not speak up.

Even with encouragement, some people simply cannot speak up. When this happens, it is important to review simultaneous lifelines that influence you now.

Perhaps you spent time in hiding. Or you were abused for your words. There are as many possibilities as there are unique individuals. What is important for you now is to understand where you are and what you need to do to create balance.

When you are a natural introvert, you suffer from loneliness, isolation, and abandonment. You try to hold on to something or someone, but cannot get a grip on anything. Introverts often live in misery their entire lives, feeling unconnected to this existence and often longing to be "elsewhere." Isolation programming kicks in, emotional issues exacerbate instead of resolve. The physical body begins to shut down as a result.

If you are a natural Introvert, then there are steps that you can take to reach a place of balance inside of yourself so that you can better interact with the outside world:

- Awareness that you are an Introvert.
- Understanding that all things come from the God-Mind, including this world.
- Agree to explore the world rather than hide from it.
- Look for the positive instead of the negative.
- Release fears, concerns, doubts, and confusion up to your Oversoul and into God-Mind.
- Permeate your physical structure with Maroon for courage.

- Move your well-established center up and anchor Self into Oversoul and God-Mind.
- Make an effort to speak to others, such as store clerks, delivery people, postal clerks, etc.
- Always keep ice blue in the throat chakra, along with the Communication Archetype.
- Mix up your current environment to mix up any stagnant internal energy.
- Review the chapter on Change in my *Decoding Your Life* book.

You are the only one who can make a difference in your world. Your world is what it is as a result of your own internalized mind-pattern. Always change your inner world to change your outer world experiences.

I easily balance my Introvert Qualities with my Extrovert Qualities.

Are You an Extrovert?

- Do you feel like you have to overcompensate to make yourself noticed?
- Do you need to be the life of the party?
- Do you do things to make people notice you?
- Do you try to make everyone happy?
- Do you have vision issues, specifically not being able to see clearly up close?
- Have you had broken bones from going forward to quickly and stumbling?
- Is your physical body in great shape on the outside but not so well on the inside?
- Do you have a digestive system that does not absorb enough?

- Are you constantly hungry because you have an unfulfilled mind-pattern?
- Do you feel like you operate outside of your center?
- Do you feel like others take from you and there is nothing left for yourself?
- Do you take the time to listen to your Oversoul and God-Mind before opening your mouth?
- Do you feel like it is important for everyone to hear your opinion whether they want to hear it or not?
- Are you mentally and physically tired at the end of the day from trying so hard to please?
- Do you like your outer world to be full of hustle and bustle?
- Are you constantly on the go, often dropping into bed at night from exhaustion?
- Do you prefer to be with others rather than be alone?
- Do you arrange your schedule so you have little "alone" time?
- Are you loud so that others will notice you?
- Do you believe you are better than others?
- Do you believe your opinions are more valuable than others?
- Does your genetic lineage support Extrovert tendencies?
- What is the influence of your simultaneous existences?
- Were you an outspoken leader who demanded respect regardless if you earned it or not?

Extroverts are often extremely insecure individuals who have a need for outer attention to tell them that they are okay. They often go out of their way to help others because they need constant reassurance that they are wanted, needed, and valuable. Inside, they have many doubts about self-worth, self-esteem, and self-appreciation.

Extroverts often are active in communities and neighborhoods where they engage in visible and charitable activities so that they are often told how much they are appreciated. They may also see what you need before you need it. They control and manipulate to receive gratitude and kudos.

Most extroverts operate with positive intentions to help. For most extroverts, it is their subconscious minds that direct the outer show. This allows them to be highly intuitive so that they are in the "right place at the right time," always waiting for the spotlight to shine on him/her to fill the empty emotional cup inside.

This means that without intending to do, extroverts take on the lessons and experiences of others feeling like they can bear the weight when others cannot not. They are often efficient and may be able to do the job better, but without Oversoul direction they take on more than they are supposed to, thus creating a wheel of emptiness rather than filling their own internal cup.

To create a balance of Introvert qualities with your Extrovert qualities, here are some things that you can do:

- Observe when you are trying to grab the spotlight and how.
- Observe if others really want your help or if you are foisting your help upon them.
- Observe if you take on the burdens of others "just because you can."
- Let others be in charge even if you "can do it better."
- Allow others to make mistakes so they can learn to self-correct.
- Breathe yourself into your center so that you always have a point of inner reference.
- Mentally pull your aura back in around your body and make sure it stays there.
- Create boundaries of where you start and where you stop.

- Choose clothes without wild designs, loud prints, deferring to more subdued colors, styles, and small or no designs.
- Do not let others into your boundaries unless specifically directed to do so by your Oversoul.
- Ask your Oversoul before you open your mouth or move your body.

Learn to feel positive about yourself from within. Release the need for the approval of others. Use affirmations to enhance personal self-worth. Review the appropriate affirmations in *1,099 Daily Affirmations for Self-Change*. You created your current mind-pattern; you can therefore dismantle what you no longer need and replace it with something better.

I easily balance my Extrovert Qualities with my Introvert Qualities.

Introvert, Extrovert Affirmations

I always ask my Oversoul before I move my body or open my mouth.

I always speak up as appropriate.

I know what to say and when to say it.

I allow others the right to their own lessons.

I release the need to control and manipulate life circumstances.

I rely on the wisdom of my Oversoul and God-Mind to guide me at all times.

I trust my own inner process and self-knowing.

Introvert, Extrovert Visualization/Meditation

- Close your eyes.
- Breathe yourself in and breathe yourself out, keeping your focus at the pineal gland.

- With your mind, will your aura in close to your body.
- Place your protection around your aura so that you know where you start and where you stop.
- Mentally make a list of your Introvert Qualities. Decide what has uplifted you and what has held you back.
- With your mind, send all that you no longer need up to your Oversoul and God-Mind. With your mind, allow what you need to fill and replace the space now available.
- Mentally make a list of your Extrovert Qualities. Decide what has uplifted you and what has held you back.
- With your mind, send all that you no longer need up to your Oversoul and God-Mind. With your mind, allow what you need to fill and replace the space now available.
- Ask if there is any specific scenario that needs clearing and if so for this to appear before your inner eye.
- Review whatever comes up. Allow your inner emotions to rise to the surface so you they can be reviewed and release. In your mind, correct and balance the situation. Play it over and over again until your mind is re-set with the scenario that you pro-actively choose.
- Give thanks to your Oversoul and God-Mind for your Inner Direction resulting in Balance.
- Open your eyes, carrying the feeling, knowing, and wisdom with you 24/7.

My Introvert & Extrovert Qualities are in Perfect Balance & Harmony.

Leadership

Believe it or not, at one point in my life I was extremely shy and introverted. I never fit in with the children around me. In elementary school I had few friends because I didn't understand others my age.

Once in middle school, then junior high, I had fewer friends. Cliques formed as several schools came together. Many of my "friends" started doing drugs, drinking, partying, sleeping around, etc. I had no interest in this sort of thing. I buried my nose in my school work and metaphysical books.

By high school I was so miserable that I found a way to graduate a year early. Freedom at last...but not really. I had issues at home that I needed to escape, so I found the only way out that I knew. Marriage at 17. I broke my parents' hearts, but I needed to find my Self. They cut the strings completely. My mother disowned me and refused to speak to me for the first year that I was gone.

Tough lessons, but ones that contributed to my own inner strength. I had to depend on my Self. I became financially independent out of necessity. I worked full time, went to college full time, and did my best to maintain a relationship with my teen husband. I was born an adult. Now I was living the life.

At 19, I officially became a dairy farmer. I borrowed $50,000 to buy a herd of cows and rent 100 acres of ground. At 25, I sold that herd. The bank was paying 18% interest on the money that I earned. That went into the purchase and payments of a hay and grain farm as well as a trucking company.

And so forth. I could continue the story, but I think you understand what I am telling you. I had to support my Self. I had to be financially independent. I had to develop my leadership qualities. I became a leader of my Self out of necessity. It was not an easy road, but I learned many things:

- One of my biggest lessons was, "Where there is a will, there is a way."
- Where there was no path, I forged one.
- Where there was no opportunity, I created one.
- Whenever anyone told me "no," I figured out a way to turn that into a "yes."
- When people laughed at me for being female (which was not uncommon for the time period) I pushed through their ridicule.
- When bankers told me to send my mother in because they didn't believe I was the person in charge, I learned to stare them down and maintain my dignity.
- When I was lonely in rural America I started a metaphysical group when even the word "meditation" was considered a word straight from the devil.
- Once I make up my mind, and I *know* that I am in alignment with my Oversoul and God-Mind, nothing stops me.

My life path developed Leadership Qualities within me.

I can help others develop their own Leadership Qualities. Because I have been there, done that, and I am still doing it.

Think about your life. Have you developed your own Leadership Qualities? If so, how? If not, why not?

Be a Leader of your Self. It is the most important job that you have.

Do You Have What It Takes?

Fair

Focus

Unify

Poise

Balance

Centered

Prioritize

Flexibility

Diplomacy

Organization

Transparency

Personal Power

Resourcefulness

Unite Opposing Forces

Identify Abilities of Others

Change Course as needed

Inner Connection to Source

Ability to See through Chaos

Inner Calm amongst Outer Turbulence

Remain Steadfast in your Inner Convictions

Compromise for the Greater Common Good

Where Are You Leading Your Self?

Have you carved out a cozy little niche within your life? One that you don't want anyone to disturb? Do you have any "get up and go"? Or did it get up and leave you behind? What are you doing to be a leader of your Self? As a leader of your Self, are you a leader of others? If so, do you like the direction in which you are leading?

Do you have it within you to want to change the world? Or do you want to hide in a cave and make the world go away. If you want to change the world, this means that you want to change yourself. If you want to hide in a cave, this means you do not want to face yourself.

It is so easy to throw stones at others. About what people are or are not doing. To read the papers and cluck to yourself about the horrors that are out there. The biggest challenge you will ever face is within your own Self.

Who are you and what is your point of being? Why did you choose to be here at this moment in time and space? Are you here to notice what is going on or to make a difference? Are you taking advantage of the End Times scenarios or running from them? What is the value of your existence if you ignore why you are here?

Are you making yourself the strongest person that you know how? How are you exercising your brain? Your body? Your morals? Your ethics? Are you supportive of yourself and your own goals? What are your goals? Do you have any? Do you use age as an excuse… I'm too young; I'm too old? Or your health? Or this or that? Can you step back, view yourself objectively and say, "Wow, I'm doing my best." Income is inconsequential…whether you make $10/hour or $1000/hour. Are you doing your best? Are you putting your best foot forward?

Do you have a work ethic? Are you a productive member of society? If you left your physical body today, would you feel satisfied that you have done your best? Do you feel like you have left some strings untied; some relationships broken; anyone who you harmed or undermined? Can you live with yourself and your decisions? Are you comfortable with who you are and what you have done? Are you at peace within yourself?

Sitting alone in your room complaining is so, so, easy. Lonely. Isolating. Detrimental to your own health and well-being on all levels. But easy.

Are you a risk-taker? What happens if someone laughs at you? Can you get through it to the other side? Does your opinion of your Self rest solely on the reactions of others? What if an entire crowd laughs at you? Can you still maintain your integrity? Can you be the sole individual who surpasses amongst the many who are caught up in the entrapment of the group-mind?

You have a lot of knowledge. Are you applying it? Knowledge not utilized is wasted. Are you wasting your time here or making every second count?

Are you part of the problem or part of the solution?

Can you step up to the challenge?

Can you take inventory of your own leadership qualities and attributes to determine what you have within you; what you are utilizing, and what is atrophying? Do you want to go through this again or do you want to do it correctly in this lifeline and be done with it?

Are you extending your hand in some way to others to help them up the evolutionary ladder or are you too frightened by what others might think?

Are you a visionary in name-only or in practice?

Are you willing to step out of your comfort zone to fulfill your obligation of creating?

Are you creating positively or negatively?

Are you a leader of your Self?

If so, where you are you leading your Self to?

Are you proud of where you are headed?

Simply by being, others are influenced and enhanced. Others will follow your example. Maybe slowly at first, but eventually they will pick up the pace. Think of your own growth. Remember how you progressed. Have patience and compassion for others, the same as you would wish others to have for you.

There are so many purposefully planted hidden pitfalls and traps that navigating these minefields; mindfields is a challenge for those who know about them. What about those without this knowledge? How will they ever find their way out without you?

Each person is here for a reason; for a purpose. While you are here, the more you can accomplish, the more your soul-personality grows. Do what you can for your Self, but in the process, lend a hand to those on the rung of the ladder below you.

The stronger you become, the stronger the path you create for the collective group-mind to follow…when it is ready.

You have so much to offer. You must be in charge of your Self. You must lead your Self out of all bondage, deeper into the positive aspects of Self. Be the best Leader that you can, and you will know exactly where to go, when to go and how to go.

A Leader Must Be Able To…

- Be lonely at times.
- Endure the jealousies of others.
- Stand firm in your own belief systems while others pick you apart from head to toe and back again.
- Be the surrogate upon which others displace their inner furies against father, mother, siblings, teachers, colleagues, friends.
- Effectively communicate your ideas.
- Identify the strengths of your team—including your own Internal Team.
- Identify inner and outer weaknesses so that you can fortify them.
- Motivate others to action.
- Recognize your power and not abuse it.
- Empower those around you.
- Understand that everyone is expendable, even you.
- Admit the error of your own ways.
- Walk through your own Internal Doubts, Fears, and Confusion.
- Pat yourself on the back for your accomplishments.

- Uplift yourself when no one else will do it for you.
- Believe in your Self and your own innate abilities.
- Know how to Persevere against the odds.
- Recognize the Source of your Inner Strength; Knowledge; Wisdom; and Courage.
- Answer "Yes" to this question:

After reading this list, are you willing to be a Leader?

Leadership Affirmations

I lead my Self out of isolation and depression.

I lead my Self out of mind-controlled oppression.

I lead my Self into positive action.

I lead my Self into a Proactive, Creative Life.

I lead my Self deeper into my Oversoul and God-Mind.

I can lead others if necessary.

I can follow others if necessary.

Leading Your Self Out of Programming

What happens when the entire world is mind-controlled and programmed? How do you live in such a world, maintaining your sanity? How do you lead others out of the darkness of their own minds when they do not even recognize the darkness? How do you lead others out when your own darkness is still a mystery to you?

How do you withstand the scrutiny of those who fear your light? First, you have to not fear your own light. Rather than close down the brilliant, shining, beautiful totality of your own soul-personality, you have to be confident enough in your own abilities to let yourself shine. You may feel like a round peg in a square hole, but it is time to stop this nonsense, succumbing to the dictates of the masses. Yes, know your audience but at the same time start taking those baby steps out of the closet in which you have enclosed yourself.

Yes, you are going to make a few people uncomfortable. This is their issue. Yes, some people will leave your life because you will no longer have matching archetypes. As they leave, others will enter. New reflections for the new parts of your Self that you are allowing Out at long last.

Rather than fear your own light, embrace it. Be prepared, because you can now see into the dark corners of Self that you have methodically avoided. Gather your strength from your light. Look into the dark corners as you release the need to be triggered and/or activated.

You can only be triggered and/or activated if you allow it. You must look through the programming to find your true Identity. Because your true identity has programming hooked into it, you may believe that you are what your programming tells you. You may act it out or become activated by it.

As long as you keep that Brown Merger Archetype at the pineal gland 24/7, you cannot be pulled into your programming. You may slip into it, but the moment you have conscious awareness of that archetype, or begin looking for it, or have the inner strength to put it back there, you have something to hang onto. That archetype keeps you together against all odds.

When you no longer fear your light, you will no longer fear your dark. The need for triggering and activations automatically leaves you. You can look at all aspects of Self without judgment or criticism, knowing that everything exists within the God-mind.

What kind of world do you have around yourself? Is it harmonious and beautiful or full of strife, sabotage and subterfuge? Which lifestyle builds more character? As much as you may crave harmony and beauty, the seedier side of life seems to be more attractive and more interesting to you.

Perhaps this is because you entered into this reality on the Holy Trinity side and so you are interested in exploring the part of God-Mind that you are not. To understand it without getting caught up in it can be a challenge.

You may squirm in your chair as you read about the seedier side of life, yet it still fascinates and intrigues. The depths to which humankind can sink fascinates. Murder, mayhem, and torment are great attention getters. These subjects fill the news. You read the details. A part of you craves more. There is a dark side full of intrigue that hypnotizes and mesmerizes every person.

This is why people love horror movies and seek other vicarious thrills. Temptation to explore the unknown. Or, perhaps the known that you are leaving behind. Put in a little toe to test the experience. Then, the experience becomes normal and eventually the abnormal becomes normal.

In this way, the frequencies that permeate society literally twist and turn the masses into a seething group of mindless, programmed robots ready to be activated with a flip of a switch. Who's going to flip that switch and how, you never really know. But the one thing you do know is how to lead yourself out of programming. You have the tools, so when that switch is flipped you do not become an activated, mindless robot...unless you choose this path.

In the short term, mindlessness is the easiest path. You can stop thinking for yourself; listen to the orders from others. You think this takes away your own responsibility for action. You simply obey commands. You stop the struggle. You relax into the groundswell of the masses. You put yourself in reverse. You release the Individualized Consciousness in favor of Group Consciousness. Time stands still as you are pulled further into the abyss.

The seedier side of life becomes your normal. The realm of the Unholy Trinity. Explore, distract, suck you in. In addition, ELF bombardment and radionic imprinting of specific frequencies are designed to vacuum the lifeblood out of you.

At one time, wine and ale were foods. Fermented foods full of enzymes to promote digestion, kill parasites, destroy bacteria. Today, wine and ale are radioncially targeted and filled with imprints designed to create addiction within you.

Pornography, gambling, drugs, you name it. All radionically imprinted to draw you in. Anything, any way to grab control over you, your pocketbook, your mind, your life, your soul.

To lead yourself out of any type of programming, you have to first decide you don't want it. You have to determine what has control over you. Nothing and no one should be in control except *you.*

You are the captain of your ship. If anyone else or anything is controlling you, then you have abdicated your position and you must take responsibility for your actions. Take back your power. Stand up for yourself. Use the affirmations provided. You have the tools; you have no excuse not to use them.

You *are* a Leader or your mind-pattern would not have attracted this issue of this newsletter to you. You must begin to change the pattern of this reality by changing the frequency in which you, personally, reside.

All change must come from within. Lead your own frequency and the rest will automatically follow. There is no time left to "think about it." The time is now. Choose wisely, otherwise it could be too late. Look at what happened to so many people in Japan. Emotionally suppressed and overwhelmed. Now they are in a reactive position. Do your best to remain Proactive in your life.

Do not wait for the triggers and activations to happen to you. Dig them out now. Immediately. Lead your Self out of mass and/or individually programmed mind-control. Set the precedence. Turn the tide. Be part of the solution, not the problem. You have heard these sayings myriad of times. Now is the time to answer the call to action.

Be your own Inspiration. Make a list of anything/anyone/any situation that controls you. How long is your list? What and who is on it? Well, guess what. If there is even one thing on that list, then you have within you the frequency that allows your Self to be controlled. Release it, regardless of what it is. Set up the mind-pattern for total Self-control under the direction of your Oversoul and God-Mind.

Lead your Self out of programming. Take care of your own life.

Understand others with compassion. Turn the programming frequency away. This takes a Powerful Person. I believe in You. I need you to believe in You as strongly as I do. Now, get busy. There is work to do.

Call To Leadership Visualization

- Close your eyes and breathe in through the top of your head, up to your Oversoul and up into God-Mind.
- Verify that your outer protection is in place: violet bubble with mirror on the outside; ultimate protection archetype; violet bubble layered with silver and then with gold, Golden Winged Lions/White Winged Lions. Whatever form of protection you prefer to use.
- At the pineal gland, look to be sure the Brown Merger Archetype is in place.
- Breathe yourself into your center.
- With your mind, call all aspects of your leadership qualities to the forefront.
- Visualize them marching into the Brown Merger Archetype. Pulling together for the greater good.
- All negative leadership aspects march right into the Brown Merger Archetype, continuing up into your Oversoul and God-Mind.
- All Positive Leadership Aspects March into the Brown Merger Archetype where the blend together to strengthen the totality of the active portions of the soul-personality.
- Feel all Leadership Aspects of Self blending, melding and growing into something bigger and better.
- Feel each cell waking up to establish its own True Potential.
- Take a look at those aspects of Self that need leading. Take inner inventory.

- Feel your inner resolve grow.
- Know that the weak areas are ready to be fortified.
- Feel your strengths growing increasingly more cohesive, coming together to Lead you into the most beneficial way of life.
- Know that whatever happens in the outside world, you are calm, centered and connected.
- Your Leadership qualities are always in direct awareness of what you need to do, how you need to do it, and when.
- Mentally affirm:

I call forth all my Leadership aspects, releasing those that I no longer need up to my Oversoul and into God-Mind; merging with all that I do need. I trust the process that is in direct awareness with my Oversoul and God-Mind. My Leadership aspects lead me where I need to be in the way that I need to be, when I need to be. I allow my high moral and ethical standards to permeate all my thoughts, words, and deeds.

- Hold these thoughts and the images that come with them as long as you like.
- Open your eyes and make some written comments in your Meditation Journal.
- Mentally repeat this "Call to Leadership" Visualization as often as necessary. Be your own best cheerleader. Support your Self on its journey. You are the best one for the job!

I AM the Leader of My Self.

Motivation

What motivates you? This is a question I have pondered for quite some time as I observe this world in which we all live.

I think of my own father, who has now lived over 90 years. He went to work at a gas station when he was 12. His father, my grandfather, used to brag that my dad "didn't cost him a cent after he was 12 years old." He was proud of my dad's "accomplishment" but of course, my dad resented this. My dad had to buy his own clothes, school books and even bought his own bed. My grandfather wanted him to pay rent and contribute to the family for the food he ate. My dad grew up really quickly. He had to take responsibility for himself because he did not have a choice.

At 12, Stewart's grandmother was sent by herself across Europe to Germany where she caught a boat to the U.S., never to see her parents again.

My maternal grandfather became the "man" of his family at 12 years old when his father died. He had to quit school and work to support his family. He lived a hard life, going on to have six children of his own who he pushed to the limit so that, in his opinion, they would never have to go cold or hungry as he had when he was growing up.

Would these things happen today? Never. At least not in North America. This would most definitely be called "child abuse."

Personally, I cannot imagine or condone this, either. However, I think we have now gone to the extreme.

A lot has changed in the past few generations.

I see so many young people not beginning to grow up and take responsibility until 30 or 35 years old. Some never mature.

I was babysitting at 12 years old. I spent the summers of years 14 and 15 babysitting fulltime for a working mother on my street. At 16, I was employed by a fabric store. At 17, I began supporting myself fulltime. At 19, I was self-employed and supplemented with odd jobs when I had to, from cleaning nursing homes to working in an art gallery. Whenever I needed funding, I found a way to make that happen.

I never sat back and complained about not having money, no jobs available, bad economy. I was self-motivated to be responsible and take care of myself. Whatever that took. I remember going to a Sears & Roebuck mail order catalogue store three times a week with a grumpy store manager who started yelling at me each time I came in. The store was on my rounds, so I kept going back. Eight weeks later when she had an opening, guess who she thought of first? Yes, I got the job and worked there for about three years, making my way up the ladder.

I accepted whatever was in front of me. Whatever I did not like, I determined a way to change it. I was self-motivated and self-responsible.

What was once my block is now my stepping stone.

I coined this phrase some years back. I love this great self-motivating statement. If you feel blocked in any way, at any time, I invite you to adopt this affirmation and incorporate it into your own daily routine. Nothing stops me once I make up my mind, except my Oversoul when I need re-direction. Even then I try every route and door until I am absolutely satisfied without a doubt that I need to be on another path.

You, too, have a story; you *are* a story; a living, breathing story. You may be so accustomed to your life that you forget what you have been through. What motivates you? What gives you the "umph" to get through life?

People used to live their lives with a little fantasy via live theater, then radio, then movies, then television, then computers. Now, people have a lot of fantasy with a little bit of living.

The Fuel That Motivates

When your physical body does not feel well, you are not motivated. I really believe that most people do not have a clue as to the meaning of "health."

I once went to an older chiropractor who told me a story about himself and his wife before he became a chiropractor. They both went to a chiropractor when they were younger. He felt great and his wife complained of a dozen aches and pains. The chiropractor took x-rays of both spines and then put them up side by side. One was twisted and obviously out of alignment. The other looked relatively straight and in good shape.

The husband automatically assumed the best x-ray was his, as he was without complaint and the other belonged to his wife. But, guess what? The best x-ray belonged to his wife. Because she was so close to alignment she felt every single little nuance that was out of alignment. She was in touch with her body.

The husband was out of touch with his body, so he did not realize how out of alignment he truly was. This was an eye-opener for him.

This is a great indicator about how out of touch most people are with their bodies. You do not even know if you are hungry or full. You eat for entertainment, for relaxation, for emotional fulfillment. How often do you eat to feed your body? Do you know what makes your body feel nourished?

Your stomach may change its message to you from "empty" to "full," but do you listen to the rest of your body? Are your lungs nourished? Your heart? Your liver? Your spleen? Your bones? Your brain? Your eyes? and so forth? Do you automatically assume a full stomach equals a nourished body?

I watched a news show about woman who weighs over 700 pounds. When asked about her eating patterns she replied that she often went until mid-afternoon without eating. Then she "suddenly" became famished and she would "overeat." So, how can a 700-pound person *ever* get "hungry"? That is what fat is about—stored nutrition. Well, her body is obviously storing something, but not useable nutrients because otherwise when she was hungry the nutrients stored in the fat would automatically be released to take care of the hunger.

As a species, humanity has lost and is losing the ability to know the physical body. What it needs, when it needs, how it needs. The only thing you are aware of these days is your stomach. When this one organ speaks to you, fill it up. It does not matter with what. Put something in the stomach and it is quiet.

Once your stomach is full, then you need to look at the rest of the body. You need to become acquainted with every organ and system of your body. You don't have to be a medical practitioner to do this.

Mentally explore the chakra bands and everything therein. Allow your consciousness to resonate with the correct color, tone, and archetypes that each band contains. Get to know the physical body that is your home. You are here for a reason. You have a physical body so you can fulfill your mission. Create the best one that you possibly can.

Stop listening to the garbage that is being perpetuated by the mass media. I read the "women's magazines" when I am out and about to keep my finger on the pulse of what is being proliferated to the masses. Talk about disinformation. Fear. Low self-worth. Focus on the negative: weight loss/gain, relationships, household decorating…and the latest meds…with an occasional success story to keep you "hoping."

Stop hoping and go within. People parrot magazines, talk show hosts, and what everyone else says. Say what *you* know, not what others know. Know by knowing. Know your own health and nutrition needs. Get to know your physical body. Your physical body, your vehicle is as important in this reality as your mind. When your body feels well, you feel motivated!

Get intimate; get deep; spend time. Dump the junk food to dump the junk mental food. Listen to your body. Let your stomach get empty so you can listen to other body parts. What does your liver say? Your pancreas? Your brain? Know how to feed the entire physical body.

My "Healthy Living" podcasts give you ideas and starting places. But you are responsible for the finishing places. Not me, or anyone else. You. Go into those chakra bands. Determine for yourself and life becomes so much simpler. The confusion goes away. The doubt. Allow Truth to resonate within you. Truth is who and what you are; refuse to let anyone tell you any differently.

You already know. Get the physical in order so that you return to your place of Personal Power—the fuel that Motivates.

De-Motivators

Life can become so routine that you often are not even aware of the "de-motivating" factors of your life.

You wake up each morning, go through your morning routine, another day, back to bed and then start over again. Sometimes I think I wake up and go to sleep with hardly anything in between!

Part of the purpose of this reality is to get you to activate your potential –to push you into the possibilities that are in your head…and then beyond, into even more than you may consciously ever imagine.

The Global Handlers look for frequencies that are "different"; moving away from the herd or "pack" mentality. When you actively move or change, you are targeted for harder control. Every single tiny hole in your auric field is utilized.

If you take over-the-counter medications, these create holes in your auric field, specifically your pineal gland. Prescription and illegal drugs loosen your chakra bands so that they are not buttoned in so tightly.

Media instills fear, powerlessness, hopelessness. Aggression, anger, resentment, and even hate.

All of this leads to subtle levels of depression. The weights on your shoulders are heavy. Gravity on Earth is a reflection of your inner burdens. Mental and emotional weights distract you.

Physical illness or discomfort. Aging. Relationship issues. Career issues. The list goes on and on. When you put this all together you understand the challenges some days of finding the place within you that is still motivated to grow! To become bigger, better, stronger when it seems that the odds are stacked against you.

In your myopic world, this is what everything seems. But the truth is that you allow all of these burdens so that you can build more muscle. Get stronger. Bigger. Better. Strong enough muscles to push these weights off your shoulders and back to Source.

There is a game of sorts going on. After all, this is a reality of duality. Which side will win? The oppressor who throws the burdens on you, or you, the potential victim, who must constantly throw the burdens off?

One after another, you are pounded relentlessly. Sometimes you wonder how much more you can take…and then another pounding when you are sure you cannot withstand even one more burden the weight of a hair.

But, each time, you get up. You get going. You make everything work. And, because you carry so many burdens you are accustomed to the weight. One by one. Hair by hair. Breath by breath. Each one does not seem to weigh much so you forget how much weight you actually carry.

This can be reflected in the physical body. If your body has gained physical weight through the years, think about how this happened. Ounce by ounce. You did not feel these ounces. You carried the additional weight easily. But now, you have on an extra 10 or 20 pounds. How did it get there?

If today, I gave you a bag weighing 10 or 20 pounds, told you to strap it on and carry it around for a few days, you would feel this weight very quickly. If, every day I took off one ounce you would not feel a great difference in your burdens. But, after a few days, suddenly you would notice that your load is lighter.

This is the same for your mental and emotional issues. For your depression. For the heaviness of your Earthly journey. How the insidious Global Handlers take control over your mind without you even realizing this. They take away your motivation to be something bigger and grander so that they can oppress. That is the game. You play their game because you do not know that there even is a game. Once you know the game, the next step is to determine if you are going to play.

Now you must make conscious choices. You know who, why, what, and how.

You must determine what is yours and what is not. What you have accepted that does not belong to you. You have to locate your own inner spark so that you can fan the flame until you recognize that roaring internal Life Force that is connected to the Greatest Force of All.

Nothing can hold you back. You are determined and unstoppable. Your outer world exists because it shows you who and what you are. When that outer picture no longer fits, you smash through that mold to create a New Outer Picture.

Every thought you think creates something. Every thought you think moves energy somewhere. What thoughts are you moving around and what are you creating? You may be de-motivated, but you are still creating something. Time to change. "Grab the bull by the horns." Banish all De-motivators from your life!

Motivators

Someone once told me, "if you never tasted a red apple, you think a green apple is really great." This statement refers to the life of most people. Most people become complacent, and therefore accept green apples. Most people have either forgotten about red apples, or perhaps never even known that they exist.

Now that you remember that red apples exist, it is your time to strive for them—the ripe, delicious apples, sweet with juices that run down your chin with each bite. Yes, you can have the best apples available. But to this, you must put the best mental food available into your mind.

You cannot expect to keep doing the same thing every day with the same thoughts and have your life turn out different. You cannot sit around waiting for someone to save you or for this or that to happen. You must take action now. You must firmly and authoritatively take control of your life.

When you are driving a car, have you ever been tail-gaited? Someone is in a hurry, so they ride your bumper, trying to make you nervous so you do what they want? You are still in control of that car. You do not let anyone push you around while you are driving. The same with your life.

You are in control. You have a lot of things riding on your bumper, trying to control you. But, you are still in control. They can only control you if you choose to let them. Take control of your life. Determine what motivates you and why. When guests come over do you make an extra effort to clean your home? Why does it take guests to motivate you? Self-motivation means you clean your home simply because you want a clean environment.

Does ill health motivate you? Or the threat of ill health? So you do the "right things" but for the "wrong reason"? You need to take care of you simply because you respect and love your own body enough that you want it to be the most wonderful vehicle you can make it while you are here. Do the "correct things" for the "correct reason" and better yet, at the "correct time."

What motivates you? What starts your heart singing? Do you allow joy, happiness, playfulness into your life? Or are you too busy filling your head space with morose and deprecating thoughts about your life? Or the nonsense that is proliferated via the media?

You are the only one who lives in your head. If you fill your thoughts with negativity, your motivation factor is most definitely going on a downhill ride to nowhere.

What motivates you to throw the weights off your shoulders? Get back into your personal power. Start over. For example, when you were a child, what did you want to be when you grew up?

Did you change? Did the dream change? or is it still there in some shape or form?

Ditch the status quo, what is expected of you and go into the career of your dreams. Want to own a restaurant? Bake cupcakes. Sell them at your local farmer's market or area businesses.

What makes you happy? When do you feel good about yourself? Or do you feel good about yourself?

Why do you keep anything in your life if it does not make you feel good? Do you enjoy the pain? Is it time to move on? Have you self-flagellated enough? Can you take that same energy that you use to tear yourself down and use it instead to build yourself up?

Do you have any self-worth? Can you make a list as long as your arm and then some of all of your positive qualities?

What are your expectations? So you need to consider re-patterning your expectations? You have changed, but what are you doing about instilling these changes in your expectations?

Want to sell your home? Clean and paint. Freshen and enliven. Do your mental work to let it go. Call in the new owners via the Oversoul level.

Need employment? Create your own. Small business. Micro business. It does not matter as long as you start, start, start.

Do not let *anyone* tell you no. The only "No" is from your Oversoul. Other than that, it is green light ahead. Go for it. If you are driving your car and you come to a blockade, do you just sit there and moan about it for days at a time? No. You find another way to go. Same with life. No blockades too large for you to hurdle.

No from your Oversoul is another word for "Stop. Re-direct Your Path." Always remember "rejection is God's protection." There is a reason you may not understand, but trust that it is for your highest good.

Motivation. It already exists within you. You can be positively motivated or negatively motivated. You can never be "stagnant" or that is the end of the precious lifestream that you have created.

Allow your inner spark to grow. Motivate. Move you somewhere. Vertically. Do not keep repeating the same experience over and over again. That is horizontal movement. You are better than that.

Focus on the Positive. Where you want to go and how to get there. Greet the challenge. This is a chance to prove who you are. What kind of mountains you can move…or climb…or go around. Know who and what you are. Your inner resources. The depths of your Being. Into the God-Mind.

I Self-Motivate because I can.

Motivation Visualization

- Breathe your Self into your Center, up into your Oversoul and on up into God-Mind.
- With your Mind, will your aura in close to your body. Place it in a violet bubble with a mirror on the outside.
- Now you have a place where you start and where you stop. You have established your Personal Boundaries.
- You let no one and no thing into your bubble without Oversoul Permission.
- Breathe your Self and breathe your Self out.
- Feel your Self sink deeper into your center; deeper into your Oversoul; deeper into God-Mind.
- Feel the deep inner connection of your Personal Trinity: Self, Oversoul and God-Mind.
- Observe the Powerful, Vibrant, Life-Giving Force of the God-Mind.
- Observe this Force moving through the Oversoul Level and into Self.
- Observe the Force within. Is it active? Stagnant? Dynamic? Barely there or roaring and waiting for you to let it loose?

- What does this Life-Giving Force look like to you?
- Do you like what you see? Do you want more?
- Open the Pathway from your depths to your Conscious Self.
- Widen the Pathway.
- Allow this Powerful, Vibrant, Life-Giving Force to fill the corners of your Soul; every cell of your physical structure.
- Feel Movement. Feel Motivation. Feel Life-Force waiting for you to direct it.
- Breathe it into all aspects of your waiting and accepting Self.

I allow Movement.

I accept Motivation.

I guide the Powerful, Vibrant, Life-Giving Force of the God-Mind to operate in and through me as needed in every area of my Life.

I am Motivated to move forward deeper into my Life; deeper into my own Inner Resources.

I am Motivated to positively upgrade all my current life experience.

I am one with all that I need to move forward; to make my Self and circumstances more soul-fulfilling.

I breathe in all that I need; I breathe out all that I no longer need.

I hold within me 24/7 internal Motivation, powered by the Life-Giving Force of the God-Mind via my Oversoul.

For this I give thanks.

- Open your eyes when you are ready, knowing that you carry exactly what you need within you, 24/7.

Motivation Affirmations

I release the need for negative motivators.

I release all physical and environmental motivator blocks.

I allow positive motivators to propel me forward.

Self-empowerment provides my motivation fuel.

Correct timing and correct reasons motivate me.

I surround my Self with Self-motivated people.

I AM Self-motivated.

Rejuvenation

Some time ago, I received an email from a longtime friend, one of my original "Life Support Group" members—a true trusted friend for several decades now! Unbelievable! But even more unbelievable was the news that she shared—one of our original Life Support Group members is suffering from Alzheimer's and is in the final stages.

This makes me so sad. Charlotte was always vibrant and involved in life. A mother of four, master-quilter and seamstress. Church volunteer. Choir member. Children's book author. Moral, ethical, and always ready to lend a hand to anyone in need.

Once, when I was at her cabin in Northern Idaho, she gave me a bottle of grape juice for my children. Not realizing that she had helpfully loosened the cap, I proceeded to shake the bottle. To my horror, purple grape juice came splashing out all over her beautiful white rug! Patiently, she helped me clean it up without a trace of animosity.

Memories of Charlotte bring me happiness and gratitude that she was an important part of my life during many challenging times. A support system. Someone to talk to who could understand without judgment or criticism.

I shed some tears, thinking about how her physical life is ending. Is this her reward for all that she gave? To live in an assisted living home, not recognizing those she loves and who love her? Alone, caught in a self-created trap within her own mind? I thought of others I know, who also lived rich lives only to falter out at the end; sad, alone, and most often physically disabled.

What is your reward for the way you live your life? You may struggle from day to day, but are you doing your best to live a moral and ethical life; a life of which you can be proud? Are you rewarding yourself along the way?

My ex-stepmother-in-law also passed away from Alzheimer's. She was a school teacher and a farmer. She worked hard. Land values went up. She passed away with money in the bank. But she did not enjoy it as she went along. Instead, it was spent on healthcare in her final days.

It is sad that you do not get rewarded with better health and a happier life. Instead, you are expected to go downhill, disintegrating back into nothingness. You are supposed to plan for this. You are taught about youth, middle age, and old age. You are supposed to prepare for a time when you will be useless and helpless. People have come to expect this. Perhaps to even secretly relish a time when you have an excuse to do nothing. And be taken care of.

What happened to the times when people lived for hundreds of years? What about rejuvenation and regeneration? Is the body leading the mind? Or is the mind leading the body? What choice are you making for yourself at this moment?

If you read everything that is written about Health, you will be busy 24/7 taking care of your body. But what about your mind? Do not put the cart before the horse. Time to put the players in their rightful positions. The horse goes first, pulling the cart. The horse is your mind. The cart is your physical body.

Your Mind is the most important tool you have. You Mind sets the scenario for absolutely everything that happens in your life. You can sit around, whining and complaining, or even simply ignoring, your inner state of being. Regardless, you are creating, creating, creating every moment in time.

As long as you are creating, learn to create in conscious awareness. Look in that mirror every single morning and affirm:

I rejuvenate, rebuild, restructure, regenerate, recharge, and re-wire my body, mind, and soul.

I exist within the Divine Perfection of the God-Mind.

Feel the frequency of each and every word upon each cell of your being. Understand the totality of your own soul-personality and how it already resonates in perfection in the God-Mind frequency. As a microcosm of the macrocosm, you already are Total Health Wealth. Allow this frequency to express in and through you. *Always.*

Weight Gain De-Mystified

Unhappy, dissatisfied, isolated, lonely, worthless, abandoned, unloved, victim. How do these words make you feel? Depressed? Downtrodden? Heavy? Absolutely! Burdens to bear that weigh you down. Emotionally you feel this; mentally you justify these feelings; physically, your body outpictures this for you.

The psychic energy that runs your physical body responds to the heaviness you feel. Your psychic energy slows down, enhancing the lethargy that emanates from your mind-pattern. You become tired, listless, bored.

You pick at foods that mirror back how you feel. You choose foods that try to fill the empty emotional recesses within. You revert back to self-survival modalities. Shelter, clothing...and of course, food. You must survive. You agree to stay here. Even if you do not want to be here. You survive and trudge onward.

Food anchors you into this reality. You ingest the frequencies that comprise the Earth Plane. Food frequencies anchor and tie your physical body into and to the physical world. In addition, each frequency has a specific color, archetype and tone that also resonates with the area where your physical body is located. As you know, color, archetype and tone create this physical world.

The food industry is designed to hold you in non-serving mind-patterns. If you eat chocolate, you ingest such things as "Guilty Pleasure" and "Sinfully Delicious." You ingest the frequencies of "Guilt" and "Sin." Both are radionically imprinted into the food that you eat. These frequencies feed and enhance the frequencies that already exist within. No one forces you. You consciously and willfully choose to ingest these frequencies.

The "Health" industry now can sell you a plethora of gimmicks. First, make you feel bad, then "try" to make you feel good. "Kiss me, smack me" programming. You know this one quite well. This is why it works.

You buy their pills, diet plans, and exercise equipment; books, magazines, and health retreats. Millions and billions of dollars are spent every year on these gimmicks. After all, you want to look great to the outer world. But no matter how great you look, you still have to deal with what is inside of you.

Here are some clues to the mind-patterns that hold your weight.

- Buttocks—holding on to what is "behind" you
- Stomach—not being able to digest life experiences
- Legs—trying to step into the future while walking through the past
- Back—support system
- Shoulders—carrying burdens
- Arms—Holding onto the negative
- Hands—grasping at…well, what *are* you grasping at that you do not think you can hold onto?

Ultimately, it is not what you put in your mouth that determines your weight—it is what you put in your Mind.

When you change your eating patterns, you force the Mind to think differently. You can only lose excess weight when the mind is ready to let the excess mind-patterns go that created it in the first place. That's a challenge for most people. Most people enjoy their issues, even when they complain that they do not.

Old mind-patterns are the comfort zone. It is what you know. When you release the old, you have to replace it with something new. Herein lies the next level of discomfort. You do not belong in the past, you are not comfortable with the present, yet the next level is unfamiliar. Taking that leap of faith is one of the most challenging steps ever. Your programming tells you not to do it. Oversoul and God-Mind cheer you on to move forward.

You have forgotten your True Self and the Magnificence of your Own Being. You deserve to Know Yourself in your True State. Start with the Mind. Magnify the Most Brilliant Aspects of Yourself that you can possibly envision. Then walk into that Brilliance. Embrace it. Allow the Brilliance to Embrace You.

Violet, silver, gold, Self, Oversoul, God-Mind. The most Powerful Combination in Existence. And it is Already Yours. Take back your own existence. *Now.* Reclaim Your Rightful Place. Walk Tall, Proud and with Dignity. Re-invest in the Human Race by Investing in Your own Soul-Personality.

When you really decide once and for all that you are ready to let go of your physical weight, the first place you start is your Mind. Release your Mental Weight and you are on your weigh—oops, I mean "way!"

Low Carbohydrate Body Cleansing

To support your mental work, you may choose to follow a low carbohydrate eating plan. I have many excellent and extremely tasty recipes online in my "Healthy Living" podcasts.

Benefits:

- Lost weight, even when not consciously restricting calories
- Improved triglycerides
- Reduced blood sugar
- Increased "good" cholesterol
- Improved insulin sensitivity
- Decreased blood pressure
- Improved energy

- Diminished sweet cravings
- Improved mental concentration
- Decreased emotional eating
- Improved dental health
- Decreased joint and muscle pain
- Fewer headaches
- Diminished PMS
- Lessened heartburn
- Improved skin

Most eating plans stop once your outer weight is gone. But remember, you must also continue to improve and rejuvenate your internal organs. Fasting, which I have discussed at length in my webinars, is an excellent form of detoxification. In fact, when done correctly, fasting detoxes the mind, which means the body automatically follows. How easy is that?

The Secret of Health Wealth

You may think such things as:

"I would be healthy if I had the money for this or that."

"I would take better care of myself if I had more time."

"I would exercise if there was a gym nearby."

"I will probably get this or that health condition because it runs in my family."

"I'm this old so I can expect this or that to start happening soon."

The secret of Health Wealth is extremely simple. The secret is so easy that most people overlook it. Some even consider it so boring and dull that they discard it looking for something fancy. The secret is so obvious that few people give it credibility.

The secret is…start where you are. If you do not have the money for something that has caught your eye, consider yourself fortunate. "Rejection is God's Protection." I learned this a long time ago from a friend and it is now one of my best companion statements. When things turn out differently than I expect, I may have a little hissy fit along the way, but I hold onto this statement to see me through to the other side.

If you do not have the money for something, then it is not for you. Or, you are not ready for it. If you do not have the money for what you "really" want, then focus on what you do have. Because this is exactly where you need to start. Where you are. A step at a time. When you finally reach where you thought wanted to be, you will realize why you needed the route you took. You have specific lessons designed by you, for you.

There are a lot of things out there to distract you. Your "lack of money" is your guide to show you what to do, where to go, and how to get there. Lack of money slows you down. Lack of money forces you into your creative side. Lack of money allows your resourcefulness to open in new and exciting ways. Lack of money creates your path. Lack of money makes you evaluate your place in life. Lack of money means you have to think differently to achieve your goals.

People who get money who are not ready for money experience some really terrific challenges. Lottery winners are easy examples. One man gave his granddaughter so much money that she became involved in drugs and was killed. Ask him now if he still wishes he had won the lottery. You know what his answer is. These types of stories are endless if you want to do your research. Do not "jump from the frying pan into the fire," as my dad would say. You are where you are for a reason. Start with where you are. When things do not go as *you* plan, there is always a reason. Observe the signposts and learn.

When you spend your money you want to maximize the use of your funds; i.e., get the most "bang for your buck" as the old saying goes. Body, mind, emotions and soul need to be in perfect alignment. Often times what you think you want turns out to be something you didn't expect. You may be jumping ahead to Step 26 when you need to be perfecting Step 8. Not having the funds slows you down.

You may feel that you are in a race against time, but in True Reality there is no time. If you were supposed to be "there" instead of "here," you would be. Release whatever it is you think you need. Ask your Oversoul to direct you to what you do need. Yes, you may be disappointed but let that go. Negative attachment to anything holds you there like glue.

Negative attachment is the cloud that hides ELF bombardments, self-sabotage, and victim-mentality. Know that there is a better plan. Once you release the old way of thinking, a new way presents itself. This is that Leap of Faith again. One door closes and another one opens. Tell, and even yell if necessary, your Oversoul to show you the door and you will walk through. Make this your mantra 24/7 until you have its attention, fully focused, and poised to move forward in the best possible way for you.

Time is an elusive factor. A minute is not always a minute. Having a great time? A minute passes in the blink of an eye. Having a really horrid time? A minute is a loooooong time. Know that you have the time to take care of yourself. Start with one minute, or five minutes. Set the imprinting of doing something. Right now.

Every day, do the same thing for one minute. Or five minutes. Slowly increase what you are doing every day by one or two minutes. Next thing you know, you have carved some time out of your day that you can use to take care of yourself. Set small goals that create the imprinting of "success." A success mind-pattern takes you a long way in all of your life. You begin to realize that time is elastic.

You do not need a gym to exercise. You do not need a large space. You can do simple stretching exercises. Can you touch your toes? Hang from your waist every day for a few seconds. Notice I did not say, "try to touch your toes." I said "hang." That is it. Simply hang. Loosen up; feel some flexibility back into your body. Nothing tough or too challenging. Simply hang. Flexible body, flexible mind. Mind is most important; Mind leads. Body follows.

Simple strengthening exercises are next. Pick up a couple of handheld weights. One or two pounds each. Hold them at shoulder height and them above your head. Hold them at shoulder height and then push them away from you keeping your arms parallel to the ground. Hold them at shoulder height and then bring them together in front of your chest. Hold them at your side and then push them back behind you. Do each exercise two to three times. Then repeat. Increase each one as you feel guided.

You can walk. You can go up and down stairs. You can run. But you do need to move. Move your body, move your Mind. Move your Mind, move your Life.

Health conditions run in families because mind-patterns run in families. Why do you think you were attracted to your family in the first place? You had to have a matching mind-pattern, whether you like your family or not. This is your opportunity to break the cycle and surpass.

Yes, it may be easier for you to take on a specific condition when it runs in your family. Every health condition exists because of mind-pattern. Mind leads, body follows. You know the health condition; you know the mind-pattern that runs in your family. You can succumb to it if you wish. Easily. This means you know a potential weak area of your mind. Correct the mind, correct the body.

Conventional medicine has a list of what you can expect. Which body parts to fail at what age. You can accept this cart pulling your horse, or you can get yourself in order, put your horse in front of that cart and refuse to participate in the brainwashing that conventional medicine would have you accept. There is a lot to be said about being young at heart. A joyous, happy, contented outlook on life precedes a cellular structure that is in harmony and peace…which translates into a healthy physical body.

Envision yourself how you would like to look. Hold that vision in your mind. Allow this vision to be refined as you move through your journey. Use the strength of your thoughts to create the physical outpicturing of your mental and emotional health. Your soul is ageless. When you truly know this within, the physical body pictures it without.

Mind is Master of Your Body

Whatever your challenges, the solution is nearby. You are never given more than you can bear. And, there is never anything that is "incurable." How many times have you heard of people who were told they would never walk again, and they did? What did they do differently than the next person? What inner motivators propelled them to disregard their diagnosis to the point of negating it entirely?

Your Mind is Master of Your Body. If you took on a burden then you have the wherewithal to unburden yourself. You feel pushed to your limits so that you can push through those limits. You position yourself for Success on a new level by reaching new inner heights. Or, you can give up, give in, and acquiesce to whatever outer control you perceive.

Some people get exhausted. They let go. They have simply had enough. This is their right. No one need judge or criticize them for their actions. Sometimes, that is the way it is. You must retreat for rest and replenishment. Then, try again. Your Mind continues to devise ways to push you through until the goal is accomplished. If not this way, then that way. You have a mission. Sooner or later, you will accomplish it. Where there is a will, there is a way.

Look at the plant kingdom, as an example. Stinging nettles have spikes with acid that penetrate your skin causing a throbbing, hot painful rash. However, yellow dock usually grows nearby which can ease the pain of a nettle rash by crushing the leaves and rubbing them into the skin. Jewelweed often grows near poison ivy and poison oak. All you have to do is slice the stem and rub it on the contaminated area to alleviate the symptoms. There is a natural order to the universe that with proper study you can observe and utilize to your benefit.

There is a natural order to your own internal universe. You are in the process of exploring and understanding that order. If you have a burden, you have a solution. Always remember that your Mind is Master of Your Body.

Your words make a difference, each one transforming your cellular structure as you speak and think.

Health Wealth is already yours. Bring it into fruition. Imprint your consciousness with:

My Mind is Master of My Body.

REJUVENATION AFFIRMATIONS

My mind as my most important tool.

I release old, debilitating mind-patterns.

I am flexible in my thinking and thus in my physical body.

I elevate and upgrade my body, mind, soul.

I flood every cell of my being with medium green to oxygenate and emotionally heal.

I am happy, healthy, whole, and complete.

I am in a constant state of rejuvenation.

X REVERSE IMPRINTING X

Ages 0–9

You learn the average age a human lives.

Brown X out those numbers.

Violet X infinity.

Ages 10–19

New Beginnings of your entry into adulthood.

Brown X Negative New Beginnings.

Violet X Positive New Beginnings.

Ages 20–29

The decade of Duality; Learning about Positives and Negatives.

Brown X Negative Imprintings.

Violet X Positive Imprintings.

Ages 30–39

The decade of Perfection.

What mind-patterns did you perfect? Positive or Negative?

Brown X Perfected Negative Mind-Patterns.

Violet X Perfected Positive Mind-Pattern.

Ages 40–49

The decade of Physical Reality. Your direction in life settles in.

Brown X Negative Life Direction.

Violet X Positive Life Direction.

Ages 50–59

The decade of Healing.

Brown X Negative Health.

Violet X Positive Health.

Ages 60–69

The decade to End any Series of Cycles.

Brown X Negative Series of Cycles.

Violet X Positive New Series of Cycles.

Ages 70–79

The decade to Complete Your Life Work.

Brown X Negative Life Work.

Violet X Positive Life Work.

Ages 80–89

The decade for Conscious Oversoul Connection.

Brown X Illusions of Separation from Source.

Violet X Conscious Oversoul Connection.

Ages 90–99

The Decade for Ending Cycles.

Brown X Physical Transition.

Violet X Physical Rejuvenation and Expansion

Ages 100+

The Decade of New Beginnings.

Brown X Negative Life Expectancy.

Violet X Living Storehouse of Knowledge & Wisdom.

Expand Your Mind, Expand Your Life

Walk on Water
Bi-locate
Pull resources from the air
Pass through walls
Move through other dimensions
View energetic imprints everywhere
Perfect physical body
Surpass physical death
Deflect unfriendly solid objects
Instantaneously travel
Levitate

Rejuvenation Visualization

- Close your eyes and breathe in through the top of your head, up to your Oversoul, up into God-Mind.
- Breathe in medium green throughout your entire cellular system to oxygenate, rejuvenate, restructure, rebuild, and rewire every cell of your being.
- Flood every cell of your being with medium green.
- As the medium green pours into your cellular structure, visualize all that you no longer need leaving the cellular structure, passing up through the top of your head, and back to your Oversoul and God-Mind.
- Above your head visualize a Golden Aleph, the archetype for God-Mind. On top of the Golden Aleph, place the archetype for Intelligent Being: Vertical Medium Green Frequency Line with a Medium Green Dot above that.
- Place everything in a Medium Green Circle.
- Within the Circle, visualize your name in brown block letters.
- Mentally state:

I now merge with the Perfection of the God-Mind. As I merge with the Perfection of the God-Mind I release into It all my Self ideas of imperfection. I am one with the Perfection of the God-Mind.

- Hold this image as long as you like. Release everything up to your Oversoul and back into God-Mind.
- Open your eyes.
- Touch back into this whenever you feel guided to do so.

My Physical Body Reflects the Agelessness of My Soul.

Relationship Healings

Have you ever had a relationship crisis? You feel emotionally distressed; upset; cannot eat; cannot sleep; tears flow. Maybe you did not see it coming. Someone who you thought would always be there for you; the kind of person who stands by you through thick and thin. The person who you felt knew you inside and out; a steady presence.

When these kinds of situations happen, they throw you into inner turmoil. You do not want to let the person go, yet here you are at a fork in the road.

How many times has this happened to you? Someone you knew or depended upon suddenly threw a few jabs at you before disappearing into the sunset? How did you feel at the time? How do you feel now? Have you been able to move through it or do you still think about "what if"?

Life is full of shake-ups and shake-outs. At the time, relationship break-ups can devastate. You have to change. You have to think another way. Process experiences differently. You are consciously forced into change. Even positive change is a challenge for most people.

You are now free to find a new level of support. The other person is now free to find what is better for him/her. The other person may have painful lessons waiting on his/her chosen fork. Lessons that do not involve you. You may want to spare that person these lessons, but you must love that person enough to let him/her go.

You no longer have matching archetypes. You probably have not for a while. When you are accustomed to communicating often with each other, you most likely do not notice subtle changes as you near the fork in the road.

Love your Self enough to move along on your journey. Trust the new road to take you to a better place. Filled with the people who are now able to understand and support you. You deserve this. You deserve the best support system that this reality has to offer.

Release and let go of anyone who holds you back; who challenges your right to reach and actualize your full potential. Refuse to allow anyone to anchor you into a repetitive past. You know better now. You have tools. You have a path. You have goals.

Thank the person for being a part of your life and for what you shared, both positive and negative. Review the parts of your Self that person represented. Understand why he/she no longer reflects you.

Rather than a relationship crisis, think of your experience as a Relationship Healing. A healing of your own relationship with your Self. A releasing of the parts of Self that no longer serve a purpose back to your Oversoul; back to God-Mind. You are never alone.

You always have YOU.

The Secret of Relationship Wealth

Relationships are one of the trickiest aspects of life. Because it is a challenge to see yourself exactly as you are, your mind-patterns attract others who mirror your reflection back to you. This concept may challenge you.

You probably first start thinking about all of those people who you do not like; those who irritate, annoy, frustrate, and generally make your life miserable. You can probably make a long list of people with these attributes. Determining what part of you these people represent may take some extra effort. You may not even be able to figure this out on your own—this is where I can help you.

- Do not judge or criticize who you are. When you judge and criticize yourself, then you do the same to others. Releasing this inner behavior releases the outer reflections. Your relationships no longer judge and criticize you.
- Accept that you are who you are because of the experiences you have been through. This means that you are okay exactly as you are. Your relationships reflect this status back to you.
- Refuse to carry guilt. Negative past actions are negative past action. You didn't know any better at the time. You did the best that you cold with what you knew. This relieves anyone trying to control you with guilt.
- Apologies via the Oversoul level to anyone who you feel needs to be apologized to. Apologize to yourself. Apologize to your Oversoul and God-Mind. Now those in your relationships can apologize to you.
- "Negative" people are teachers. Each one of these people took time out of his/her life to show you something about yourself. Your mind-pattern brought them to you. Thank them. This opens the door for others to appreciate and thank you.
- Be your own teacher. Understand the lessons you bring to yourself. Make a commitment to greet your self-devised challenges. Now, your relationships can understand and commit to you.

If you were supposed to be off on a desert island somewhere, you would be. You are here, with people because this is exactly where you need to be with whom you need to be.

Every relationship is about *you*. The Secret to Relationship Wealth is a Healthy Relationship with the most fascinating person you know—*you!*

Unlocking The Secret to Creating the Relationships You Want

Unlocking the Secret to Creating the Relationships You Want begins with your initial mind-pattern imprinting by your initial caregivers. This initial imprinting replicates in your relationships. This includes everyone from friends, colleagues, and neighbors to teachers, clerks and government officials. You play out the same scenarios over and over again. Same people, different names. Same song, different verse.

To help you understand, read through the list below. If this happened to you, or a parental figure treated you this way, then there is a common result.

- Adopted: Abandonment
- Berated: Shame
- Emotionally Distant: Isolation
- Force-Fed: Not wanting to be here
- Ignored: Needy
- Helpless: Unsupported
- Hungry: Unable to nurture or receive nourishment
- Negative Father: Male issues
- Negative Mother: Female issues
- Parent Death or Abandonment: Unlovable
- Physically Beaten: Seek Punishment
- Powerless: Voiceless
- Sexually Abused: Failure to Connect to Others
- Suppressed: Introverted
- Verbally Abused: Low Self-Worth

Many people run away from their families. They have negative experiences in childhood that carry forward into adulthood. Some people even change their names. However, frequency is frequency. Your mind-pattern matched the mind-pattern (color, tone and archetype) of your parents at the moment of conception. This is why they are your parents.

What were their mind-patterns? What was yours? Why did you choose them? If you chose them, why do you run from them? What can they teach you? Do they still "push your buttons"? Can you be around them without getting caught up in their drama?

If you cannot deal with the mind-patterns that a brought you here, then you are destined to replicate them throughout all your relationships. Did you feel overpowered by your Mother? Then you will attract females who try to overpower you. Or, males with the characteristics of your mother who do the same thing.

Did your father stand by while your mother overpowered you? You will attract males who will continually not be there for you. You may have left your family, but your family has not left you. You simply recreate your initial imprinting scenarios. You fill the slots with different people, but the mind-patterns are the same. You replicate the same dramas except the people have different names.

If you cannot figure it out, then the lessons intensify. The situation is so "in your face" that you can no longer ignore it. Something in the mind-pattern must be corrected. Just as good can get better, bad can get worse. God-Mind does not differentiate between the two. While God-Mind is neither positive nor negative, It contains both. God-Mind is Limitless in both directions.

Generally speaking, stay with what and who you know rather than continually changing the players and scene. Allow the situation to move away from you, rather than you move away from the situation. When you have done your work, the challenging person or situation literally falls away, whether you want it to or not.

Without matching mind-patterns, no interaction takes place. This is why you might have severe issues with one person, but another person does not. No matching mind-patterns.

Mind-patterns are active. They move to the front, middle, back and everywhere in between, depending upon outer and inner activations.

If you are in a complicated relationship that you deem negative, then you need to stay there until you figure out why you attracted this in the first place. Because if you leave, you are going to attract the same person again. He/she may have a different name, but it is the same person—but maybe worse.

Of course, if you are physically abused, you need to leave. However, you need time alone. You need to recognize the mind-pattern that created this within you. Then, you need to do your release work. This can happen in an instant or it can take some time, depending upon how ingrained the mind-pattern as well as your willingness to let it go.

If all you know in your life is abuse, you are uncomfortable without it. You know how to act, react to it. You know what to say, what to think. Without it, you have to develop into another persona. This is a leap. You may not be able to traverse the chasm in one jump. You may have to build a bridge to get you across.

If you do not know how to build a bridge, you have to do research. Find the tools. Find the materials. Trial and error. Building a bridge to cross a chasm is a process. It changes you. You think differently. You react differently. The process eventually puts you on the other side. You are a different person. If you could have done it in one jump, you would have. But you did not. Because you were not there...yet.

Have patience in your impatience. You do not understand your own process. But you are getting there. When you see the end of any journey, you have less patience. If I told you it would take 20 years to build the bridge, you would sigh, resign yourself, and begin. But, when you get to year 19, you can feel, breathe, hear, see, taste the end. Impatience multiplies when you most need patience. This is where you are right now.

You are tying up many lose ends. This is why you feel impatient. You know that once you are through these specific lessons, you will not be going through them again. You feel the next layer of experience pulling you. You want to be "there" instead of "here." You must keep yourself in the present moment so that you do not lose momentum at the last second. You do not want to stop the process only to have to re-start it again, somewhere else.

Resign yourself to surpass, wherever you are, whatever your initial imprinting. Give thanks to those who provided the entryway for you into this reality; who supported the learning that you chose, whether you view it as positive or negative. Give thanks to everyone who now helps you complete these lessons.

All these people are really only you in another form. Appreciating what they offer means appreciating your Self. Understand, accepting, and yes, even loving who and what you are as well as the process that brought you to this point. Understanding the totality of you means you begin to understand the totality of the God-Mind Itself—neither positive nor negative, but containing both. It wants to know who and what It is. You are Its finger that explains this. Do not discount one second of your journey as not being equivalent to the next. If you were meant to be separate from humanity you would be.

The Holy Man does not go up the mountain because he cannot stand the people. He goes up the mountain because the people cannot stand him. His bright light forces them to see their shadows. What are your shadows? Are you as okay with them as you are with the rest of you? Do you accept *all* of you? Do you like all of you? Do you love every aspect of your own Soul?

This is The Relationship that is paramount to all others. Love your Self first; Accept your Self first; then and only then can you truly love another. Then and only then does the mind-pattern pull those to you who truly love you as a reflection of your own love for Self.

Give you to you, whole and complete, in whatever shape or form you come in. For *all* of you is a part of the God-Mind. Reject any part of *you* and you reject a part of the God-Mind. Self-acceptance, self-appreciation, self-support, self-love means the outer world can breathe a sigh of relief. Finally, this can be reflected back to you, supporting you in all endeavors, including your relationships. How true are *you* to *your* Self?

The Secret to Creating the Relationships You Want is to BE what you want.

WHO ARE YOU?

Independent: You need No One.

Dependent: You need Everyone.

Enabler: You encourage Others' Negative Behavior.

Vertical Line In Hyperspace Language: Being.

Dot In Hyperspace Language: Consciousness.

Horizontal Line In Hyperspace Language: Frequency.

Medium Green In Hyperspace Language: Emotional Balance.

Put these together and you have the Relationship Archetype.

Interdependent: You are a Conscious Being who Gives and Receives in Emotional Balance.

RELATIONSHIPS AFFIRMATIONS

I release the need to judge and criticize my Self.

I accept my Self exactly as I am.

I like who and what I am.

I love all aspects of my Self unconditionally.

I support my Self in all my learning processes.

I have a positive supportive relationship with my Self.

I now have fabulous positive supportive relationships in all areas of my life.

CHILDHOOD SURVIVAL SKILLS

How do you feel about children? Whether you have them or not is irrelevant. How you feel about children represents how you feel about yourself as a child. If you cannot deal with what happened to you as a child, most likely you will not like children.

If you did not feel tolerated, you will have a challenge tolerating children. If you have no patience for them, most likely no one had patience for you. If you feel neutral about them, then you are either ignoring your childhood feelings or you were treated with indifference. If they annoy you, then someone was annoyed with you.

Take a deep and honest look at your feelings toward children. Now, think about yourself as a child. What parts of you still reacts as a child? Does your temper easily ignite? Do you have a tendency to throw ugly words about? Do you have effective communication skills? Do you easily break into tears? Do authority figures frighten you? Do you sneak around to get what you want?

Do you have a living, breathing child within that you acquiesce to when life gets tough? Early survival skills that move forward when you don't know what to do? As a child, you could not get away. You were at the mercy of those bigger than you. You had to do what they said, regardless of how you felt. You did not have choices.

These types of experiences leave a child traumatized. Even justifiable experiences to an adult may not make sense to a child. The child does not have words, only feelings; no words to refine the feelings. Similar experiences in the adult world can trigger similar reactions. All of a sudden, you are a child again. The old feelings rise up, overcoming logic and reason. The part of you that was not allowed to express now happily tramps around releasing all the pent-up feelings of long ago.

This is how you survived. You made it. You are still here. Broken, bruised, and scarred, but nevertheless, still physically present and willing to go on. Logically, you can explain your past, but emotionally you still hurt. This affects your current relationships—most often, adversely.

Now, it is time to grow up the Child Within so that the trauma is released; so you can love and appreciate the Child that never felt loved or appreciated. As this happens, your ideas and attitudes toward children change. You can embrace their innocence as you embrace your own. You can appreciate their exploration and wonder in this reality as you now do yours. Your heart opens with compassion to the trials and tribulations of their journey—overwhelming to them but understandable to you.

Relationships improve as you now act like the adult that you are. Old mind-patterns creating negative childlike behaviors are gone. Unconditional Love for all parts of Self flood your Being, allowing others to also feel and express Unconditional Love for all parts of You. You have new survival skills—adult survival skills. You are finally in an Adult Relationship with Your Self.

Oversoul Relationship Healing Visualization

- Breathe yourself into your center.
- Out through the top of your head with your breath; up into your Oversoul and God-Mind.
- Breathe in; breathe out anchoring your Self in the strength of your Oversoul and God-Mind.
- With your eyes closed, take a look at your auric field. Notice how far it extends from your body.
- With your mind, will your auric field in close to your body.
- Surround your auric field with a violet bubble with a mirror on the outside. Now you have boundaries of where you start and where you stop.
- With your mind, create a mirror image of your Self, with the same boundaries and violet bubble.
- Place a Medium Green Vertical Line with a Dot over it within your auric field.
- Place the same within your mirror image.
- Connect the two with a Medium Green Horizontal Frequency Line.
- Feel your Relationship with Self Bond, pulling the mirror image into your Self.

- Feel your Self Whole and Complete. In Harmony and Peace with who and what you are. Where you have come from. Where you are at this moment. Where you are going.

I am whole and complete.

I AM in Harmony and Peace with who and what I am.

I heal my Relationship with My Self.

All my Relationships are now healed via the Oversoul Level.

I have a Perfect Relationship with my Self, Oversoul, and God-Mind.

All is Well is my World.

- Feel the Child Within grow up.
- Feel all that you no longer need release up to your Oversoul.
- Feel forgiveness on all levels for Self and Others in your life.
- Feel Unconditional Love for the person who you are and the people who have helped get you there.
- Know that the most important Relationship you have is with *you.*
- Give Thanks to your Oversoul and God-Mind for a Supportive Relationship.
- Open your eyes.

My Relationships Positively Support Me.

Rumors & Gossip

Whatever you give out comes back to you.

Think about this the next time that you spread a rumor, or gossip about someone. How would the other person feel if he/she knew what you were saying or writing? How would you feel if that person were standing right there beside you—would you say the same thing?

Look at the color of the sound coming out of your mouth—is it clear because your words are clean? Or is it colored with anger, bitterness, frustration, hate, maliciousness, self-righteousness, or jealousy? Do your words make a point about anything? Or do you just have a need to hear yourself speak?

Are you certain that what you are stating is true? How will you feel if you find out that you are spreading lies about someone? How do you feel about leaving yourself open so that others can spread lies about you?

Does what you say affect others on an energetic level? If the rumor/gossip is true, does it pull the targeted person up or down? Do you care about the effect your energetics have on this person? If you send out words that pull another down, what are the personal ramifications of your actions? What will your mind-pattern pull back to you?

Do you struggle enough without having to deal with others spreading rumors and gossiping about you? Do you want to have to deal with the energetic pull of others pulling you back into a mind-pattern from which you are struggling to extricate yourself?

What do you think happens to the person when you give them a derogatory nickname? Does this pull him/her up or tear him/her down? Would you like this going on behind your back? Do you think using a derogatory nickname for another person pulls *you* up or pulls *you* down?

Do you like to hear others laugh and think you are clever at the expense of someone else? When you do this, do you stop and think about who this person really is? Have you taken time to look on the Oversoul level deep inside this person to see who he/she really is rather than just make a cursory judgment/criticism, and roll with it?

Do you think spreading rumors and gossiping helps to elevate you along your own personal path? Do you ask your Oversoul for permission to speak before you open your mouth? Or do you just do whatever it is that you want to do? Once you know the law, what do you think is the ramifications for breaking it? Do you think your lessons become easier or harsher?

Do you realize that the more you know, the more responsible you are for your own actions? Are your intentions to heal the global consciousness or to destroy it? How much healing do you think that you do when spreading rumors or gossiping about others? How much more time do you think others have to spend healing in order to clean up after your actions?

If you see another person do something that you consider inappropriate, should you discuss it with others? Is it possible that there is "more to the story than meets the eye?" Do you quickly judge and/or criticize the other person? Do you take the time to look at the energetics behind the action? And, if what the person does/says *is* inappropriate, is it up to you to tell others about it? And is it *really* inappropriate on the Oversoul level, or is it simply *your* judgment call?

Sometimes if you cannot come to a conclusion with which you feel comfortable, it is appropriate to discuss it with someone for the sole purpose of uncovering the truth. Once you have the truth, then go up to your Oversoul to determine what you should do with the truth. Never make these calls yourself. And, if you are not sure what the appropriate action is even after working with your Oversoul, then give all your words and actions up to your Oversoul, asking that everything be blessed, cleaned up, and corrected as you go. Always work from the Oversoul level.

Before you speak or write about anyone for any reason, you always need to ask your Oversoul for permission to open your mouth or set your pen to paper.

If the answer is "no" but you do it anyway, there are consequences because you are now much more responsible for your actions.

When you know the correct action to take and you do the opposite, you break Universal Law.

No matter where on the path you are, you can walk off it and become so lost that it can be extremely difficult to find your back—you can set yourself up for many lifelines of struggle, heartbreak, and heartache.

The higher you are, the harder you fall.

You are never so high that you cannot fall. And, you will fall harder and your lessons will become extremely more difficult and painful.

If you are in a support group of any kind, ask your Oversoul what this group is supporting you in. A true support group is a support for your *upward* journey on the evolutionary spiral. A true support group does not hold you where you are or pull you back. You can get stuck in a hyperspace support group just the same as you can get stuck in any other support group.

Just because you are doing hyperspace techniques and someone else is not, does not make you better than the other person. It only means that you have a different way of learning. If you are doing hyperspace techniques with a group, this means that you have pulled a group of like-minded people to you who learn in a similar way. In the overall scheme of things, this is not positive or negative, it simply is. No one is ever better than anyone else. In the exploration of the totality of God-Mind, *everyone* is equal in importance.

You can destroy an energy seed, by talking, talking, talking and doing nothing, or you can nurture your energy seed by action and deed, growing it into something bigger and better. You always have a choice.

If you are not moving upward, if you are staying where you are, or if you are being pulled backward, you need to take a look at what you are doing and why, as well as how you got there. Traps are everywhere to pull you back and the only person ever responsible for your backward movement is *you. Always remember:*

Whatever you give out comes back to you.

Social Anxiety

Do crowds make you nervous? Does the thought of speaking in a group put knots in your stomach? Is speaking in front of a group practically unthinkable? Do you get "tongue-tied" in social situations and cannot think of anything to say? Do you have entire conversations in your head, but cannot seem to get the words out of your mouth?

Do you later think of what you "should have/could have" said? Do you spend time criticizing what you did manage to say? Do you think that people are watching or judging you wherever you go? Do you even avoid speaking on the telephone?

If so, then you are not alone. "Social anxiety is the third largest psychological problem in the United States today," according to the Social Phobia/Social Anxiety Association.

The bottom line for all of these situations is really lack of self-confidence and self-worth. Usually, you bring these mind-patterns in when you are born. Your environment either helps you proactively overcome the mind-pattern, or enhances your inner situation, making it increasingly difficult to effectively communicate in any social situation.

For example, did your primary caregivers encourage you to express your opinion, or were their opinions the only ones allowed to be spoken? If you are innately introverted, but are lovingly encouraged to say your inner thoughts, you create a positive and proactive way of strengthening one of your weaker attributes—that of effective communication.

If you are innately introverted and when you gather the courage to speak you are ignored, ridiculed, or punished, then you certainly are not going to venture out with your words very often. Or, if you have a natural exuberance and are a great communicator, but are ignored, ridiculed, or punished, you react to the outside world by inherently shutting yourself down.

As children, most people are encouraged to listen to the teacher, acquiescing to him/her rather than encouraged to mutually resolve personal differences. While not every teacher is this way, the system where most children spend their early childhood is designed to meet the unspoken needs of the group rather than any concerns voiced by the individual.

In addition, if you are a specifically programmed person, you are most likely programmed to not speak about your programming experiences and memories. If you do, then most often you are physically punished, with emotional and mental trauma following. This adds to a mind-pattern of isolation and further ingrains social anxieties.

In all cases, your sense of self-worth and self-confidence diminish, sometimes seemingly to the point of no return. As an adult, you most likely do not remember every incident, but most likely focus on the end result—which is your own lack of effective social interaction and your nervous to paranoid reactions.

Most people have some degree of social anxiety. For most people, regardless of background, sharing, speaking, and interacting does not automatically denote "kindness, compassion, understanding, caring, mutual challenge solving, and/or relief of emotional/physical pain." Instead, the very actions that could "save" you become the actions that torture you.

People with social anxieties perceive each time that they share, speak, or act, as an opportunity for someone to emotionally or physically hurt the, or remind them on some level of a time when this happened. The communication process or attempts thereof, remind you of your lack of worthiness to even exist. These realizations, whether consciously acknowledged or not, exacerbates the anxiety that already exists within.

People with social anxiety look for ways that people can hurt or disappoint them. Because this has been your experience, you automatically set your defenses to "high" before you determine if there is any justification for this. This does not set up the process for successful communication.

When you do try to communicate, you have your own set of filters that process whatever communication comes back to you. Most likely, somewhere between the other person's lips and your ears, their words flow through your own set of filters. What you actually hear may not be what the other person actually means to say. This is why it is important to use your Oversoul as a filter so that all your preconceived ideas on all levels are removed. This is the only way that you can truly objectively hear what the person wants you to hear. Listening through your Oversoul may not reduce the anxiety level of your "output" communication, but it can help with the "input" process.

Once the input process becomes less threatening as you hear what is really being spoken versus your filtered version, your output communication becomes less reactive. You can send your output through the Oversoul levels. This aids the other person in correctly hearing what it is you wish to communicate. All of this helps for cleaner, clearer communication that does not get muddled within life experiences that have absolutely nothing to do with the intended communication process.

There are many things that you can do to correct and balance your own personal social anxiety. First, recognize that you do have a challenge when it comes to hearing what other people actually say/mean, so learn to use the Oversoul level of communication.

Pass your fears out through the top of your head to your Oversoul. Allow it to flow and flow and flow.

Even when you use the Oversoul level, you find that some people do communicate with malice. These people become your "test." Are you worth standing up for? Can you stand up for yourself and be heard?

Before going into any social situation, be sure that you have your T-Bar Archetype balanced, your Self-Reintegration Archetype in place, your chakras in the correct color/order, and you have your protection in place. You may want to place an extra layer of brown for grounding around yourself.

Check your throat chakra to ensure that you have a good ice blue color there. Mentally wrap your throat area in maroon for courage to speak up. Make sure you do not have anything there which symbolically keeps you mentally restricted—high or buttoned collar, tie, choker-type necklace, etc. Open up the throat by wearing less restrictive clothing and/or accessories. These things do make a difference. Plus, the other person to whom you are speaking picks up on these "closed down" type of clues, similar to body language.

Realize that you are not alone—probably everyone to whom you speak has a form of social anxiety on some level, somewhere in his/her life. Use the Oversoul level to determine what is really happening, versus what your filters tell you. Also use the Oversoul to prepare everyone in advance for your conversations.

Use the correct color codes to make a difference. Think about the clothing that you wear, as well as the colors. Do they promote or close down communication? Think about the words that you choose. Recognize your own weaknesses. Then proactively push yourself a step, or a half-step, at a time, to move beyond your own self-imposed boundaries. Do your release work on those people who you perceived added to this mind-pattern, and include yourself!

Think about how you would like to be, hold the vision, use your affirmations to get yourself there, and allow your Oversoul to guide the process. Make an effort not to judge or criticize your progress, but instead observe it, let it go, and know that each time your efforts and results will improve—even if the improvement is to stop judging and criticizing yourself! You really are no different from anyone else—it is just that this is something that most people do not discuss.

No one really watches you as closely as you watch yourself. You can make a million "mistakes" and you can probably list them in detail one by one. But no one else can. You are your own harshest critic. Most other people really do not care, so do not build their view of you into something that it is not accurate. Release your need to be harsh with yourself and fill the void with the pale pink of Compassion from your Oversoul. Self-love, self-worth, self-confidence; you can do it by beginning the process *now.*

Spiritual Warrior

Do you think of yourself as a spiritual warrior? If not, then this is a title to which you might want to give some serious thought. In today's environment, the tide is against spiritual movement, much less spiritual development. The entire Earth is so heavily and thoroughly bombarded with waves and waves of ELF that the best that most spiritual seekers can hope for is to maintain the status quo.

The Global Handlers do not want you to find out any more spiritual truths than they pass out through organized, conventional religion. After studying the religions of indigenous peoples and taking their knowledge, the Global Handlers ridiculed these religions as superstitious, called the natives heathens, and turned public opinion against these peoples. This still continues to this day.

As a spiritual warrior, you must develop the mental acuity and perception to delve into spirituality in its purest form. Doing so means that you save not only yourself, but ideals and ideas that are all but extinguished as people are driven to distraction on all levels. Humankind has become mentally bereft of nourishing ideas, emotionally pulled in every direction as relationships become increasingly fragmented and distant, and physically disabled and weak as the food supply dwindles down to only merely enough real nutrients to maintain the physical structure as a shell of its potential.

As a spiritual warrior, you must be strong enough to fight to regain your lost spiritual ground. You must dive deep into your own internal waters quickly because the outer world is doing everything it can to lead you anywhere but where you can find your own personal power. There is a thick, sticky, energetic ELF soup that is layered in the atmosphere, permeating everything beneath it, from the food that you eat to the buildings where you live, work and play and into your own physical body to befuddle your brain so that your true mind can only barely function.

This is not a battle, this is a war; a war to save your own soul from further sinking into a myriad of mass confusion. You are at the mercy of the advanced technology that in the hands of a few, tricks you into believing that the technology is more powerful than your own mind; your mind that is consciously connected to your Oversoul and God-Mind, the most powerful force that can possibly exist.

As a battery with a never-ending power source, how could the Global Handlers trick you into believing that you are helpless and they are all powerful?

> Why do you live in fear of their lies and deceit?
>
> Are you not a microcosm of the macrocosm?
>
> Are you ready to stand up and claim your power?
>
> Do you clearly hear your own inner war cry that is trying to catch your attention; to force you to remember who you are and from where you come?
>
> Are you through with the distractions and pettiness of the world?
>
> Are you ready to turn the tide and reclaim the life that you designed for you?
>
> Or would you rather suffer at the hands of those who want you to feel pitiful and small?

Listen within and you will hear the still, small voice that is not so still anymore, that is crying louder and louder through your internal distractions in hopes that you can finally hear it.

Feel the heartbeat of your own internal spiritual warrior. Reclaim your right to a healthy mind, body, and soul; a whole and complete lifestyle; true knowledge and the wisdom to use it appropriately. Hear your battle cry in your effort to save yourself from going down with the ship when the ship is an illusion and the water is life-giving not life-taking.

As you develop your spiritual muscle, the oppressors will not be pleased. They will take new, more powerful action against you, forcing you into retreat. But the joke is on them, because the more they push you, the more you learn how to develop your spiritual muscle out of necessity; out of spiritual soul survival. Spiritual muscles that have lain dormant for far too long now awaken, strengthened and encouraged with each memory that finds its way into your conscious mind.

Your most challenging oppressor becomes your greatest teacher, unknowingly and unwittingly leading you to become the greatest spiritual warrior ever! Your tactics increase, your tools grow, your skills are enhanced, your spiritual muscles are exercised and nourished in ways you never would have accessed were it not for the obliging nature of the oppressors.

Stronger and stronger you become, winning back your own identity, fighting to get out of the prison into which you have willingly walked. You are a spiritual warrior! You have overcome the oppressor, because the oppressor is only a reflection of you! You have come full circle, meeting yourself where you started by lifting the lid off your own oppression and releasing the need to have your internal oppression outpictured for you and to you by others.

As the old "helpless, woe-is-me" mind-pattern dismantles, there is nothing to hold the oppressor in your space. You find that the spiritual warrior within has found true freedom at last. That which you are looking for is truly inside. Correct your own inner imbalances and the outer imbalances automatically correct themselves under Universal Law. Behold the mighty spiritual warrior! You have won the battle against yourself and in doing so, the battle in the outer world ceases to exist.

Who Is A Healer?

When the mind-pattern of a person is out of balance, all areas of a person's life are affected. Life becomes increasingly muddled, complex, and consuming. Even though it takes many weeks, months, and sometimes years for these situations to catch your attention, they usually have been building for a long time. They rarely just happen overnight. This applies to all issues, whether they are physical, mental, emotional, spiritual, career, relationship, financial, etc.

When people finally realize that they have an issue, most want a quick fix. Because these situations make them feel "bad" they want someone or something to make them feel "good"—immediately!

People choose a variety of routes to achieve this good feeling. Some people choose allopathic medicine, which suppresses the physical symptoms, or surgery, which simply cuts out the bad stuff. Some people choose legal or illegal mood-elevating drugs that promote a false sense of wellbeing.

Some people believe that if they remove specific people from their lives, that everything will be fine. Or, if they have a different job, they will be happy. Or, more money…this seems to be a great "problem solver." In the minds of most people, this "healing" that they are looking for will make them "happy" once and for all. Most people think, "if only this or that was different, I would be happy."

The majority of people are determined to find someone or something outside of themselves that will heal them or their life situation. This simply does not exist. You put yourself in a specific place in life for a reason. You did not just fall into your life. You created it one step at a time. Even if you think it was unconscious, a part of you knew exactly what was happening. This part of you allowed you to create your current circumstances. Because this part of you created your life step by step, this part of you knows how to dismantle the uncomfortable situation step by step.

Only *you* can dismantle the situation, whether it is mental or physical. Everybody and everything else is only a crutch/aid/support that ultimately can only re-direct you back inside of yourself. You got where you are by yourself, you have to get out of there by yourself. You may create support to help you move on, but only you can actually do it. This is your task; this is your mission. It may not be as grandiose an objective as you would like, but the ultimate journey truly is and only can be fulfilled by you.

You are your own guru/teacher/healer. Only you can "fix" any imbalances. If someone else comes in and does it for you, then he/she learns—not you. You may find that healing yourself is not fun or pleasant; you may find that it is a struggle. You may find people who say "let me do it for you." Let me touch you and it will go away. Let me say a magic jingle, or light candles, chant, or anything else their imaginations can come up with. That may sound more interesting to you, and more exciting to you, then you doing your own boring work. And, of course, it definitely sounds much easier than you doing it yourself!

A balanced life is not just about happiness—a balanced life is a myriad of emotions and experiences so that you enjoy the full embodiment of what this reality has to offer. Happiness is a much overrated catch-word that is not a stand-alone emotion. It needs support and grounding from a myriad of other emotions and life experiences. The garden of your life is deeply enriched by the manure that is used to fertilize it.

Stop looking for a healer to help you. Another person can help direct you to where you need to be, or help you determine how to unravel the tangle that your life has become. Sometimes you "cannot see the forest for the trees"—you are simply too close and too involved to be able to see how you got to where you are. Then, allow the strength of your mind-pattern to pull the correct information to you that helps get you through your muddle. But, no one else can do it for you. You may garner tools "here and there" but *you* are the only one that can use them. No one else can use them for you.

You may think that if you could only go somewhere else, you would be healed. Maybe you think your healer is a geographic location. While, again, this can be a crutch/aid/support, ultimately, *you* are the only one who can heal *you.*

If you allow someone or something to heal you, then you will only re-create the situation somewhere else with someone or something else. Until *you* change, nothing else truly changes. You can run, but you cannot hide anywhere. *You* are the creator and the healer.

Never put anyone on a pedestal. Everyone is always equal. If someone says that he/she can heal you, think twice, and then twice more, and if you still are not sure, you better continue your evaluation process. No one *ever* successfully heals another.

Do yourself a favor—declare yourself your own best and true healer. Gather your tools; prepare to do your work. Stay focused and maintain your Self, Oversoul, and God-Mind connection. Your path becomes narrower and also more defined. More boundaries, more rules, more success. There is nothing like triumph from within, a step at a time. These are the lessons from which you learn; these are the lessons that you remember; these are the experiences you finally and ultimately, complete. The secret to being healed is realizing who the healer really is.

Wisdom

When I was a child, "metaphysics" was not a common word. Most of the general population had never heard the term. There was even debate about the meaning of the word, which I simply defined as "meta" meaning "beyond," so metaphysics simply meant "beyond the physical."

People who used metaphysical principles were described as "metaphysicians." I liked that term and intended to apply it to my Self one day.

Most people knew the word "occult," which is rarely used these days. Why? Because occult has taken on a meaning of dark and evil. However, all occult means is "hidden." I tried to explain this to people in my early days of teaching, but this word already had connotations that discouraged anyone "not of the devil" from using it.

In the sixties, there was talk of "dawning of a New Age." This brought rebellion and the "right" of people to do what they wanted, when they wanted. This meant "Women's Liberation" which really was the start of the Androgyny Agenda—making both sexes "the same."

Free love—aka wanton sex for all as a result of birth control pills. Legalized abortion, more acceptance of mind-altering drugs and other substances, identifying who and what you are regardless of how other people felt about it—breaking up the family and long-held social norms.

As the infrastructure rules were dismantled, new rules formed to take their place. Finding your Spiritual Self was encouraged through media icons who young people eagerly emulated to the consternation of their elders. The old ways were old-fashioned and no-longer-desired standards of life. Any institution that held the family together was a candidate for destruction in its present form.

Soon the New Age was filled with psychics, astrologers, numerologists, tarot card readers, shamans, and everything in between. No one wanted to be who he/she truly was. New names, new identities, new looks. "Peace, love and light" was the mental and emotional drug that allowed people to escape personal realities, life challenges, and taking responsibility. Why look to your Self when you could spend hours gazing up at the sky waiting for the Space Brothers to fix everything, or better yet, to take you away?

I watched all of this, and more, take place in utter amazement that people could be so easily led. Personally, I made my goal to never be led. When the fashion went from pointy-toed shoes to square-toed shoes, I was the last one to change. Whatever was "in vogue" I ran the other way. I did not want a part in whatever the mass population chose to explore for the moment. I purposefully chose to not fit in.

I never had a desire to be a part of the crowd. I never liked what I saw the crowd doing. I saw the masses as loud, thoughtless, careless, and shallow. While little girls played with their Barbie dolls I was writing metaphysical lessons for children. I read books on yoga, philosophy, mysticism, health, and mental/emotional healing as well as studied metaphysical laws.

I learned to look through the vast amount of information that was proliferated throughout society to determine for my Self what was real and what was devised for distraction purposes. I never wanted to be distracted. I made a decision so long ago I cannot even tell you when, that I wanted "the straightest, shortest, most focused, most narrow path to God."

In addition, I decided that I wanted the best that this Reality has to offer—best relationships, best spiritual knowledge, best physical objects, best health, etc. I would rather take the steepest path, wait a little longer, but get what I really want at the correct time for the correct reasons.

I recognized that a lot of information was, and of course still is, available to everyone. But simply because people have access to information, does not mean that they know how to use it.

I found out that an "educated person" is not necessarily the wisest. That everyone holds deep wisdom, but not everyone can access it. I learned to look within the deepest recesses of my Self for my own Internal Wisdom. When I did not look deep enough, I was pushed.

I decided that I did not want to be known for "Peace, love, and light," even though those were the preferred qualities of the time. I wanted to be known for Wisdom.

Acquiring Wisdom has been and still is my Personal Quest. I want to share my Personal Quest with you. I love learning. I love knowledge, but most importantly, I love knowing how to use knowledge correctly.

20 Steps to Accessing Your Inner Wisdom

1. Go with your gut feeling—If something does not feel "right" most likely it is not.
2. Always question.
3. Investigate and explore.
4. Think about what others say and do, but stay with your gut feeling.
5. More people saying one thing does not make that group of people correct, even those with of like-minds.
6. Accept that not everyone can grow with you.
7. Others may be on your path for a while, but when the paths diverge, let them go.
8. Remember that there are many paths to God.
9. Stay true to yourself and your path.

10. Before making any choice, determine if you can live with yourself regardless of the outcome.
11. Make peace with yourself at the end of every day—did I do my best?
12. Make peace with your life—did I do the best with the tools that I had at the time?
13. Let go of negative "space-holders"— people, places, or things that are not growing with you.
14. Do not be tainted by the experiences of your past.
15. Forgive but do not forget the lessons.
16. Focus on vertical growth by asking new questions confirmed with new answers.
17. Be willing to move beyond your comfort zone to discover the Truth.
18. Stay true to your personal morals and principles.
19. Do your best not to add to the degradation of the world.
20. Pay attention to your "gut feeling"—Always.

Unlocking Your Inner Wisdom

A long time ago, people learned through apprenticeships. This meant that knowledge was handed down directly, person-to-person. Regardless of trade, craft, or profession, people learned directly from each other. With careful guidance, people were taught one-on-one about how to bring out the best of what he/she could do.

If you were a shoemaker, you could specialize in what kind of shoe you wanted to make. The same could be said of anyone, from warrior to healer. There was time for contemplation as you practiced and became involved with your trade, craft, or profession. Having someone talk to you directly about what you want to learn can help the process by leaps and bounds.

I always tell you to know yourself. The more you know what is inside of yourself, the more you understand what is inside of others. For example, if you were an angry person but are working your way through the process, you definitely recognize this in other people. You know the ins and outs, the intricacies of balancing this emotion. Even when someone says, "I'm not angry!" you can recognize anger in that person, even if he/she cannot. Why? You know all about anger.

The same is true of a trade, craft, or profession. When you know the details or your work, inside and out, then you can recognize in others what is within you—and beyond. Because you know where you are and where you want to go; your skills and abilities; your strengths and weaknesses; your hopes and dreams, you can recognize all of this in others.

You are an "expert" because you have spent the time studying every aspect of your outer work. If you want to go a little farther with this definition, you can say that you are an expert because you have made all of the "mistakes." Of course, you understand that mistakes are really only a redirection of your efforts from an erroneous path to a more correct one.

This simply means that you have tried many tools and methodologies. From experience you know what works and what does not work. When you pay attention to this process of trial and error you don't have to use your time repeating the same process with the same results. You can jump ahead several steps to build upon what is already known instead of repeating what has already been done only to come to the same conclusions.

When one person teaches another, and the other person actually listens, this is how humanity evolves. Now, it is extremely challenging to identify the "experts" amongst the many people who think they know, but do not.

This is how knowledge is hidden. You are distracted, entranced, and enthralled with "show," which means you stop looking before you get to any substance. You do not have anyone to tell you that you are looking at the fluff without any substance. You do not have anything to gauge what is "fluff" and what is "substance."

Society has purposefully been shaken up so that it is no longer cohesive. The process of learning from one person to another is largely lost. Societal elders are considered useless and old-fashioned; ready to put out to pasture starting about age 55 and no later than age 65. Youth has broken its link to the knowledge, experience, and Wisdom of the Elders. Youth do not want old-fashioned advice. Youth want what the media offers over what the Elders offer. They do not see through the shallowness of the fluff to see that there is no substance.

Not only is knowledge hidden this way, but so is Wisdom. People have forgotten how to live because they are not connected to each other. People are not passing knowledge from one generation to another, much less Wisdom. This disconnection is only an outer reflection of the disconnection they feel from their Source.

This is the plan, and it is working. However with awareness, you have the potential to change everything. You must feel that deep inner connection inside to your Oversoul and God-Mind. This is why the negative circumstances are so important at this current time. This is a "last ditch effort" to separate those soul-personalities who are determined to once again feel the connection to Source from those who do not.

Negative circumstances put you into a state of desperation. This means you have exhausted all current resources. When you feel like this, frightened, alone, and desperate, where do you turn? Within. Prayer. Supplication. Energetically, you dig deeper within. You *must* find new resources, or at least up-to-now untapped resources.

You fret, stew, ponder, question, plead, beg, bargain, and energetically force yourself to find some kind of knowledge that will move you somewhere, some way. All you know is that you simply *must* move. You rock and roll your inner energy, forcing your circumstances into focus. You narrow your path. You think on the issue 24/7. Focus.

Focus brings what you need before your inner eye. When you remember that everything exists in the Eternal Now, you know that the answer to your quandary already exists. Somewhere, your quandary is already resolved. All you have to do is focus through the quandary to get to the other side. Using the strength of your mind-pattern, you bring that resolution to you.

This process is your path to Inner Wisdom. Not only are you digging out the knowledge that you need, but you are learning how to use it correctly. You also must keep in mind that the process you go through is like a birth. Just as the baby is squeezed and pummeled going down the birth canal to clear and activate its body functions, so is your knowledge being squeezed and pummeled into something usable as it goes through an energetic birthing process.

Having someone with you who can show you the way is ideal, like what I do in my one-on-one work with people, from Hyperspace/Oversoul Mastermind Group to seminars, personal intensives, and personal consultations. With guidance, you bring out what you already have within you that you may not be able to see or know how to express…yet.

Plus, you learn how to use the knowledge that you access with Wisdom. This means that you know how to do what you do appropriately and correctly at all times.

Knowledge can be used for cruelty as well as to enhance. If you are on a path of garnering positive experiences, then you need the wisdom to use the knowledge appropriately. There are many wonderful people who do not know what they are doing, so they actually cause more harm than good because they lack the wisdom to know what they are doing. While their intentions are positive, results can be disastrous.

Aligning knowledge with the Wisdom to use it appropriately is an acquired ability. You have to be able to recognize when what you are doing is correct. You must go with that gut feeling that says, "Yes, move forward," or "No, stop."

How many times have you not paid attention and then found out later why you should have? You may not always know anything beyond the moment, but as long as you live each moment in the present with awareness you will know what to do in the next moment. When you trust that process of inner Wisdom to guide you, eventually you will see the entire picture.

You can call in the Frequency of Wisdom at any time. Wisdom is already in place, inherently yours. When you stop the distractions long enough to go inside; when you are willing to listen to your own inner guidance instead of outside influences, you will have unlocked and accessed True Inner Wisdom.

If you do not pay attention to the instructions of your inner Wisdom, it will shut down. If you don't use it, you lose it. A common saying with layers of meaning that can be applied to every avenue of daily living. You can choose to stumble around in the dark, filling your life with excuses, or you can get on the straight and narrow path that focuses you in on exactly what you need, when you need, with complete understanding.

Wisdom is an amazing frequency to establish in your life. With Wisdom, all things are possible. With Wisdom, all things are explainable. With Wisdom, your life broadens and deepens in personal self-satisfaction. Attaining this level of Wisdom also means making choices. Wisdom is not about taking the easy road—it is about taking the most focused road. Not everyone will want to embark on that journey with you. Continuing to rely on that inner Wisdom as your guide, you will make the correct decisions for you.

Inner Wisdom Means…

- Observation
- Understanding
- God's Timing, not my timing
- Learning from and listening to each other
- Using knowledge in accordance with Universal Law
- Using correct knowledge for the correct reason at the correct moment.

Some People…

- Do not want to use the knowledge that they have properly
- Do not want the responsibility that comes with knowledge
- Simply want what they want when they want
- Think that because they *can* do something, they have the right to do it
- Fool themselves that they are at a specific level of learning when they are not there yet
- Put on blinders, complain about their life, and are very happy in their complaints.

Because it is easier to…

- Use psychic energy than go via the Oversoul level
- Gossip than hold your tongue
- Look the other way to get what you want than use metaphysical laws
- Eat the food on your plate than wait for something more nourishing
- Rip other people apart than discriminatingly look at Self
- Be impatient than patient.

All short-term benefits with long-term consequences.

Inner Wisdom Affirmations

I unlock my Inner Wisdom.

I access and accept my Inner Wisdom.

My Inner Wisdom now pours forth into my conscious mind.

My Inner Wisdom allows me to use knowledge correctly and properly.

My Inner Wisdom instructs me wherever I go, whatever I do.

My Inner Wisdom is my Guide to All Success.

My Inner Wisdom Guides me 24/7.

Wisdom Visualization

- Close your eyes. Focus your attention at the pineal gland between the eyebrows.
- Breathe yourself in and breathe yourself out.
- With eyes closed, bring your auric field in close to your body. Surround yourself with a bubble of violet. Around that place a layer of silver and then a layer of gold.
- Breathe deep within to activate a brilliant burst of golden light; your Deep Inner Wisdom Frequency. It is already within. Now is the time to acknowledge it.
- Observe how it brightens and grows all-encompassing in and through every cell of your Being.

Deep Inner Wisdom is now active in every area of your body, mind, and soul.

Deep Inner Wisdom guides you deeper into your chosen life path. You have the knowledge. Wisdom explains to you what it means and how to use the knowledge.

Your path becomes more narrow and increasingly focused. Others may not appreciate your growth. Distractions grow exponentially.

Regardless, you stay focused on your specific path and the tasks that you came here to accomplish.

With Wisdom as your guide, you stay True to yourself and what you need to do.

Continue your self-exploration with self-awareness.

Wisdom Frequency Permeates Every Cell of My Being.

Part VIII

Reproducible Archetype Cards

Reproducible Archetype Cards

The archetypes in this book are copyright protected. However, Janet and Stewart give you permission to copy these archetypes for *your personal use only* as long as you include the Expansions copyright that is included alongside each archetype, and maintain this copyright so that Expansions continues to receive credit for its work.

Thank you for respecting this unique work presented to you by Janet and Stewart.

Archetype Cards

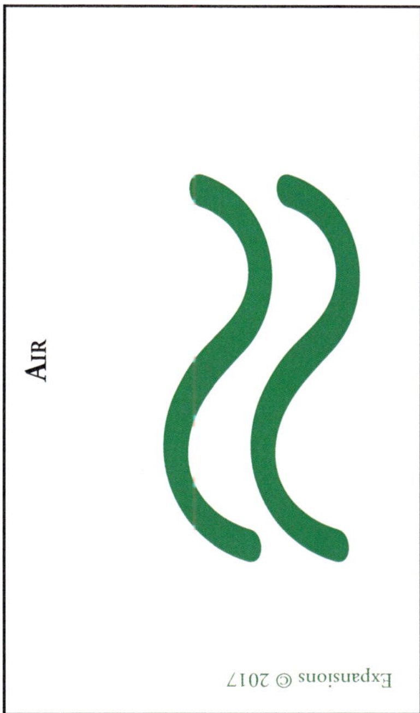
Air
Expansions © 2017

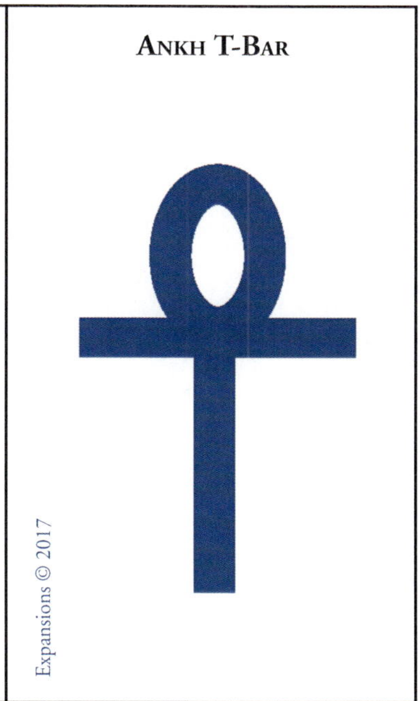
Ankh T-Bar
Expansions © 2017

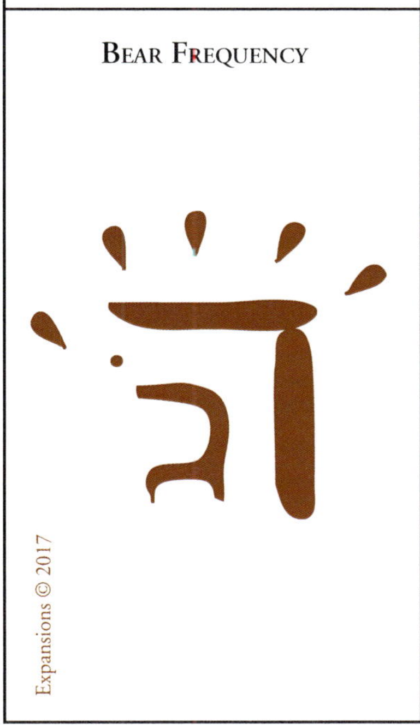
Bear Frequency
Expansions © 2017

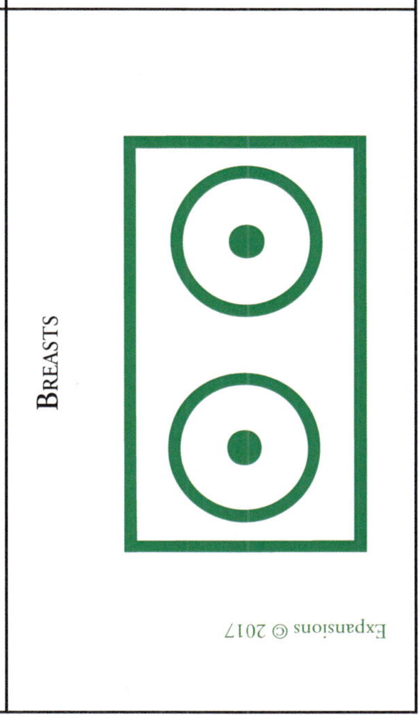
Breasts
Expansions © 2017

Cancellation

Chakra System

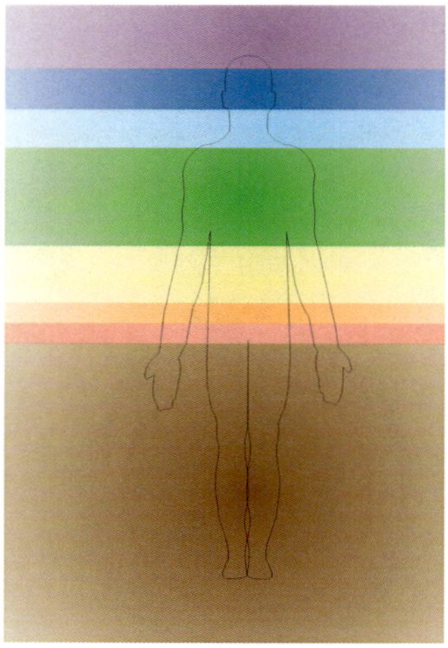

Communication

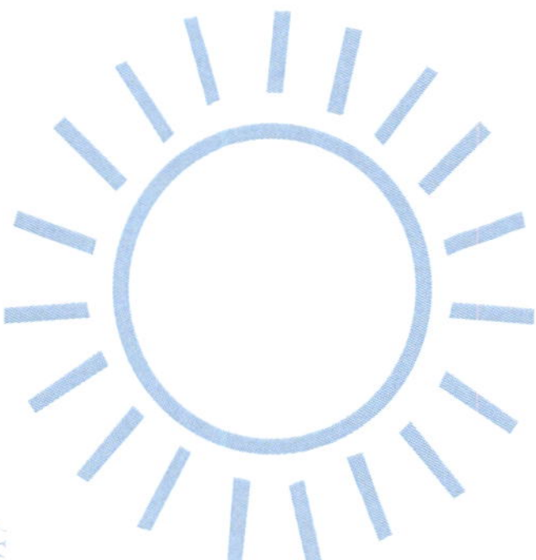

Dolphin Frequency

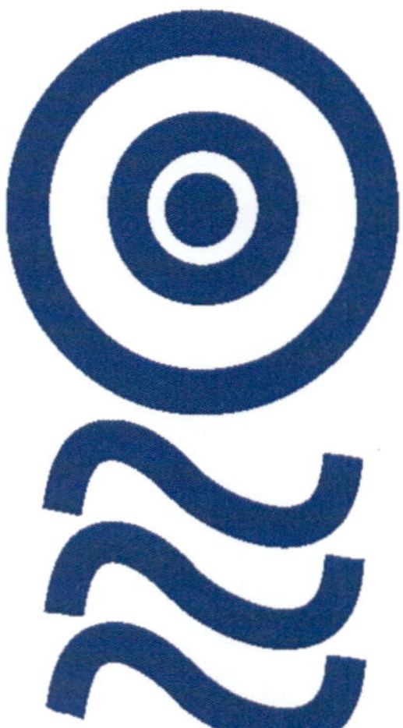

EARTH

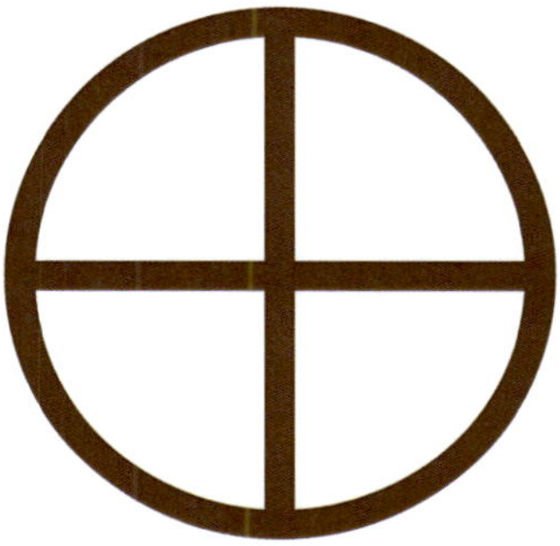

EMOTIONAL BALANCE/PINEAL GLAND

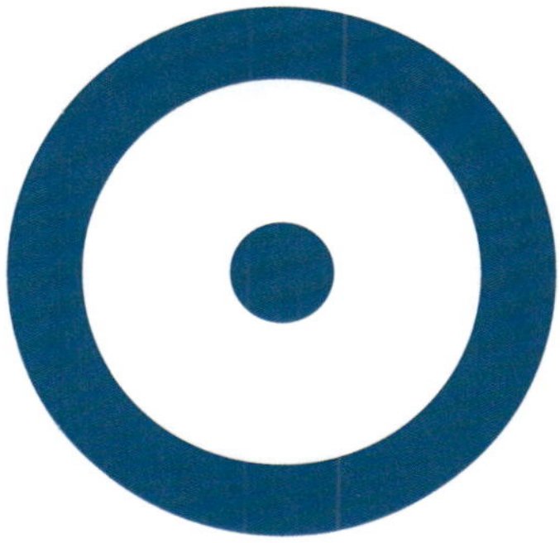

EXPANSION

FEMALE ORGASM

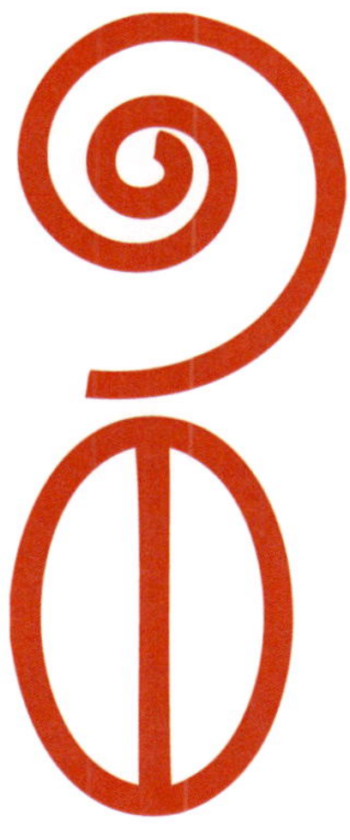

Fire

God-Mind

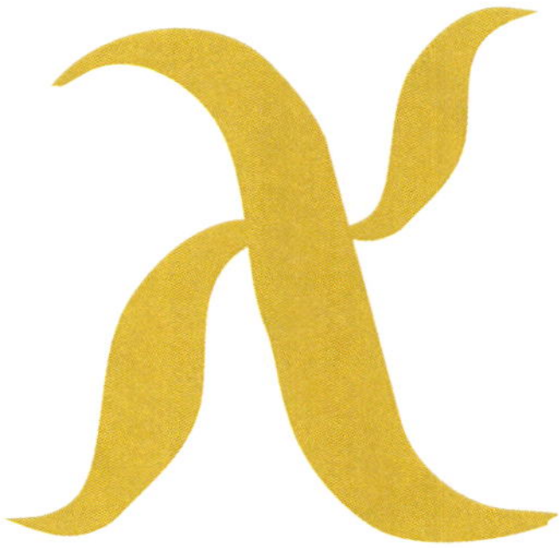

Green Psychic Flush

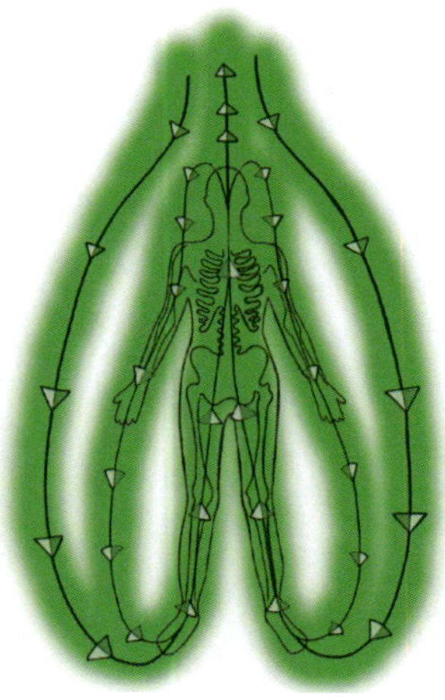

Happiness

Individualized Consciousness

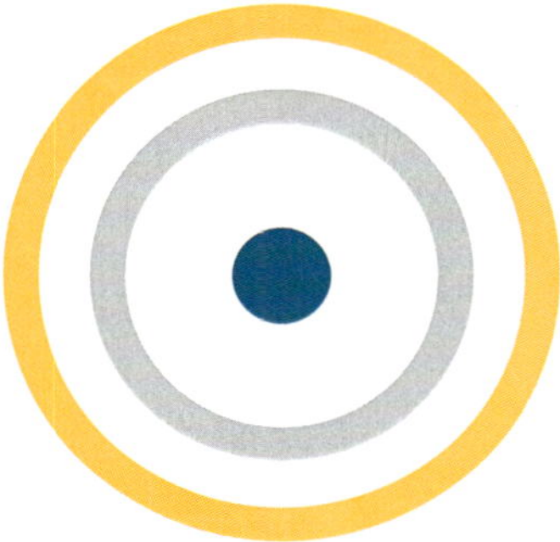

Lake

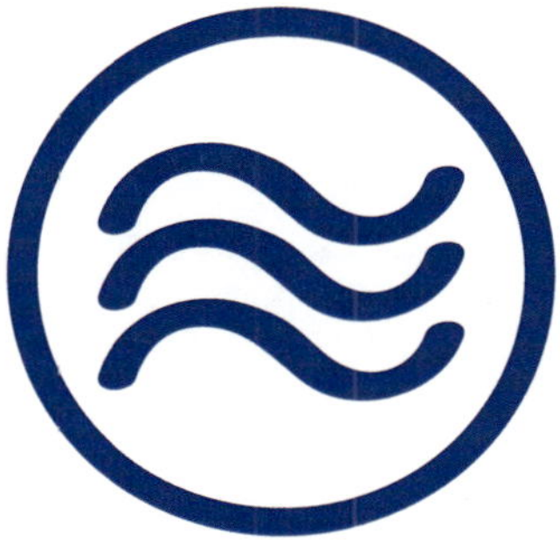

Leadership

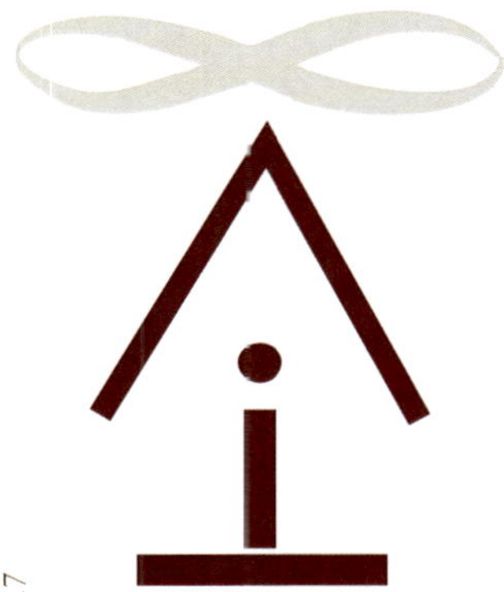

Lion Frequency

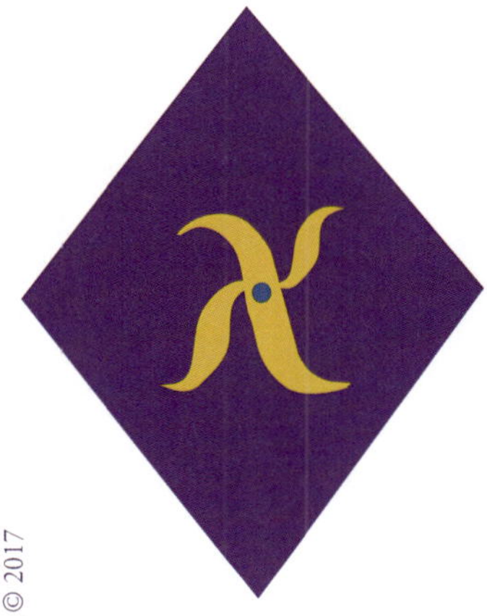

Logos Christos

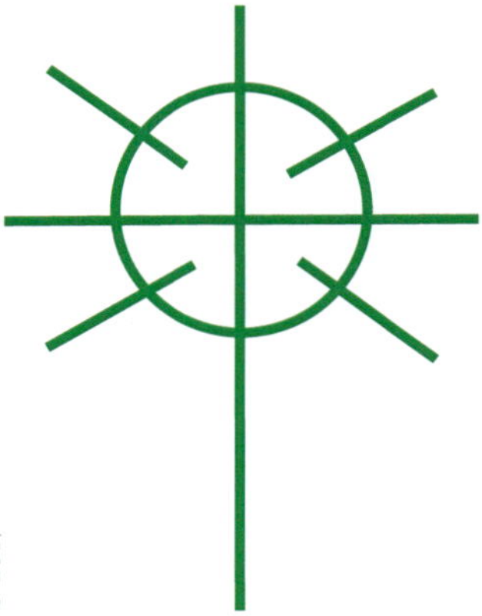

Lowercase t-bar

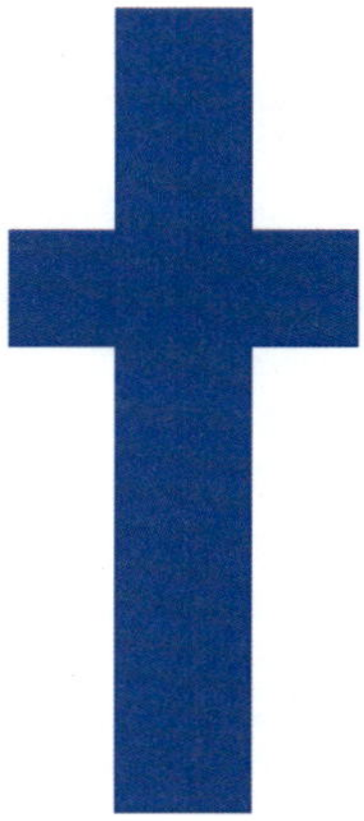

Male Orgasm

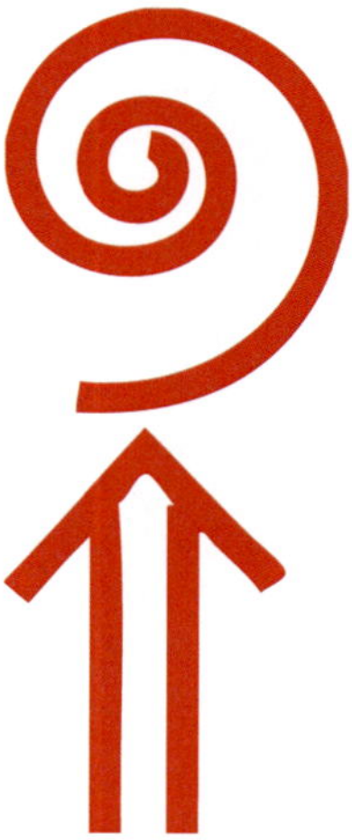

Maltese, Magdalene Cross

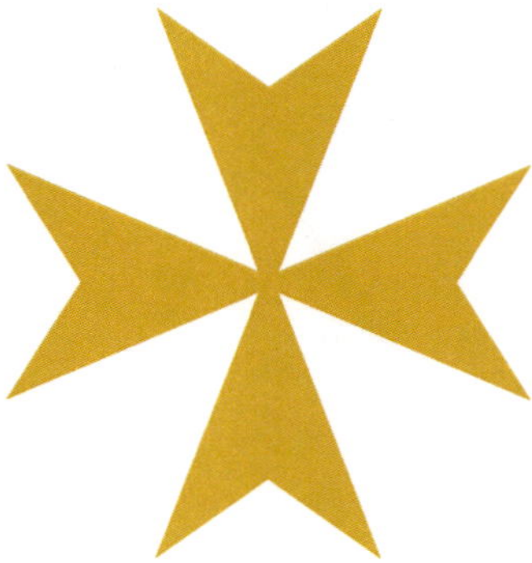

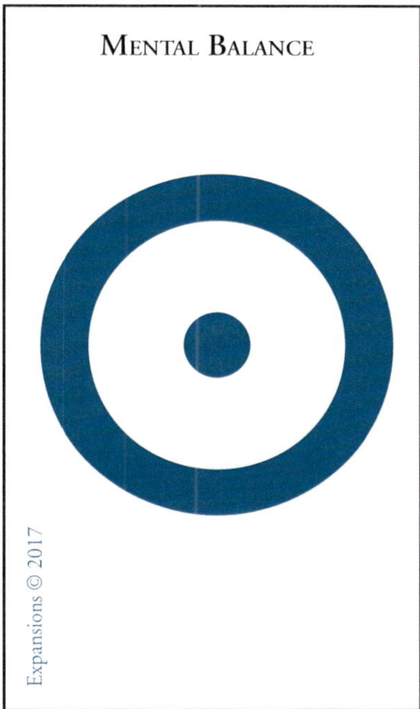
MENTAL BALANCE
Expansions © 2017

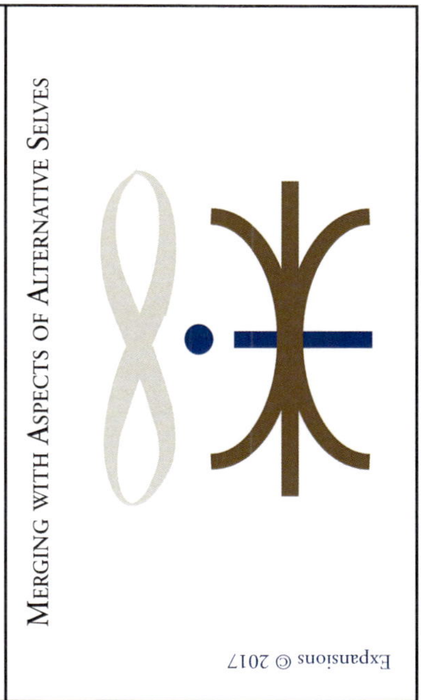
MERGING WITH ASPECTS OF ALTERNATIVE SELVES
Expansions © 2017

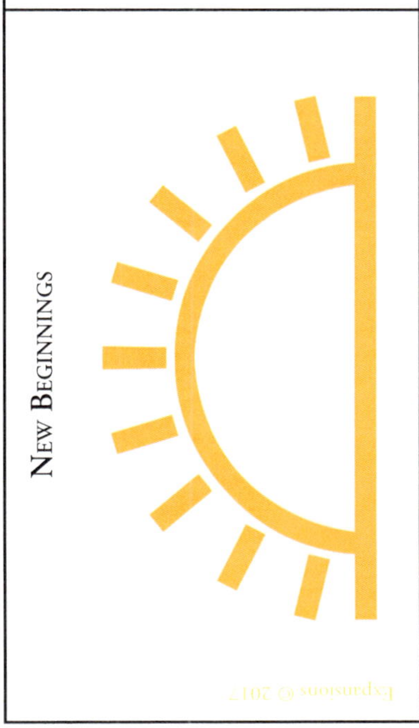
NEW BEGINNINGS
Expansions © 2017

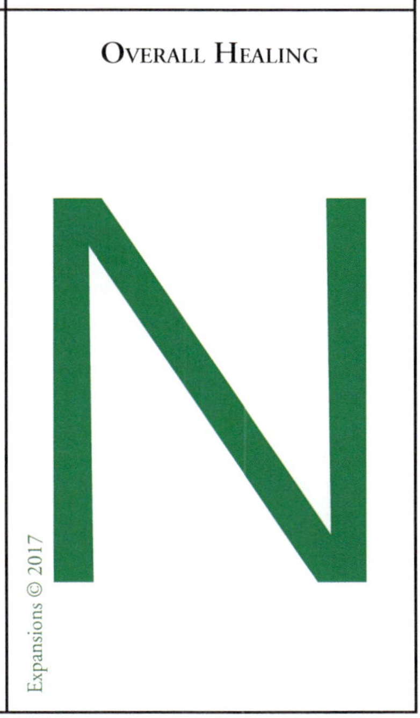
OVERALL HEALING
Expansions © 2017

OVERSOUL

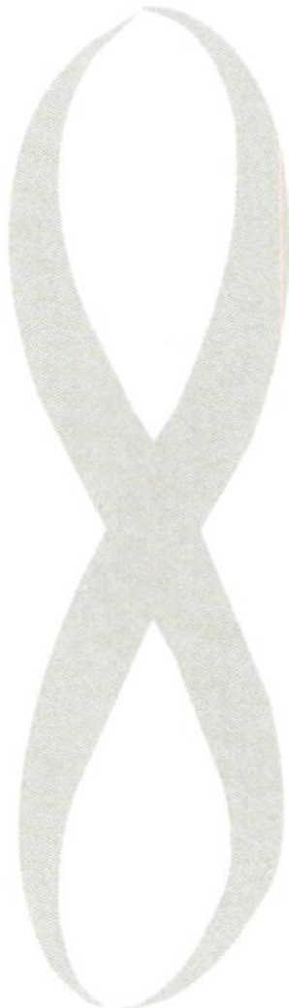

PERFECTION/
MANIFESTATION/CREATION

PI, VIOLET

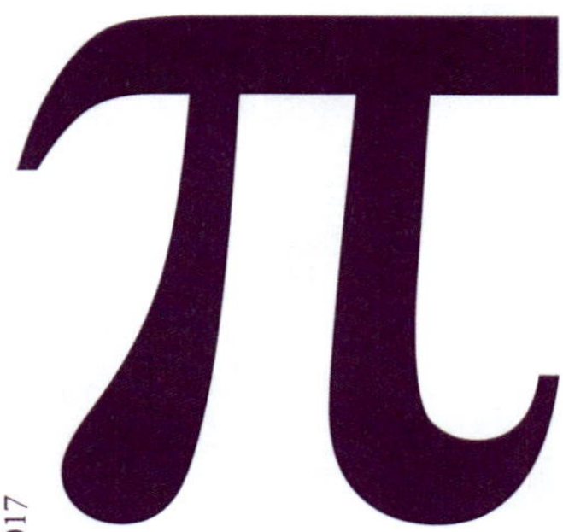

PINEAL GLAND
(EMOTIONAL BALANCE)

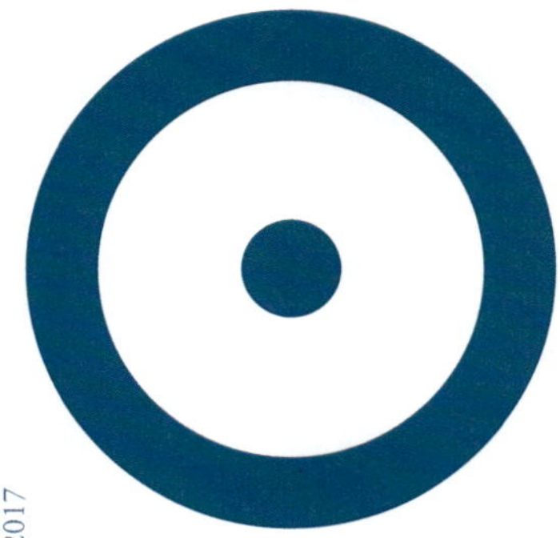

POWER

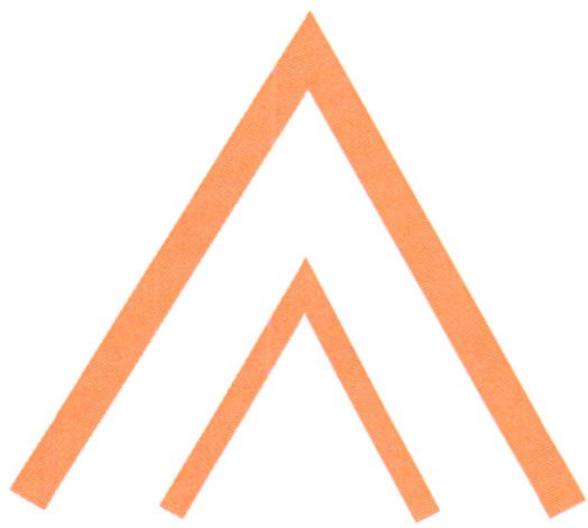

PREGNANCY

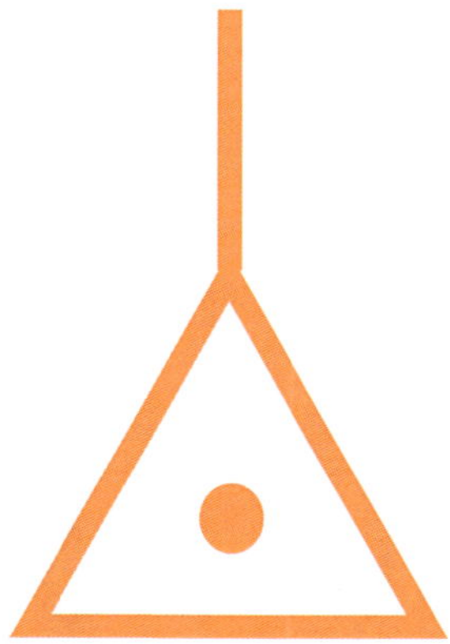

PREGNANCY PREVENTION

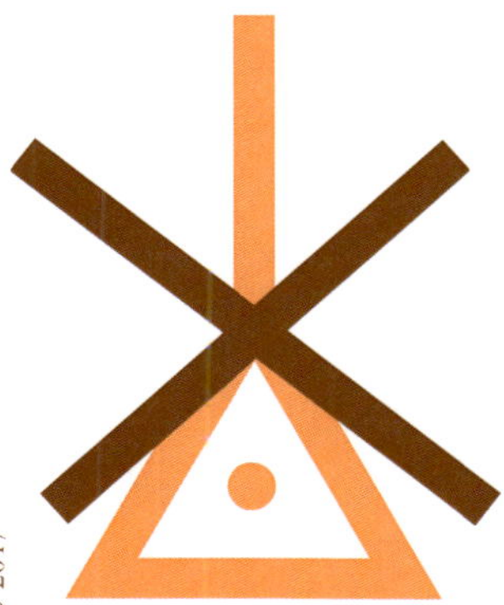

REJUVENATION

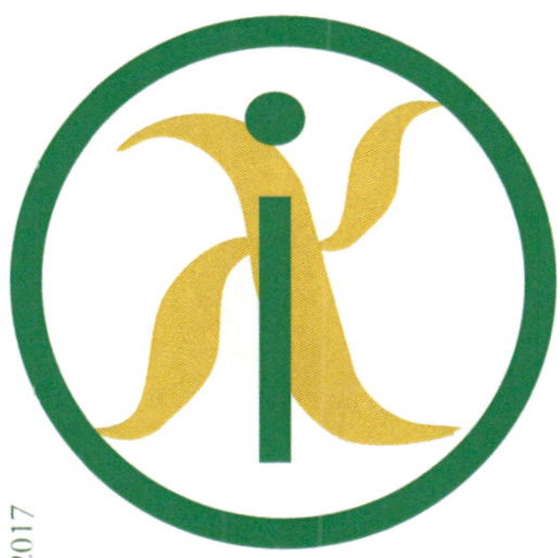

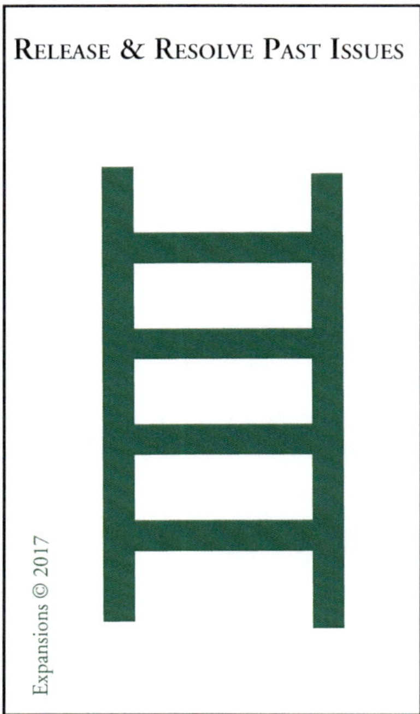
Release & Resolve Past Issues
Expansions © 2017

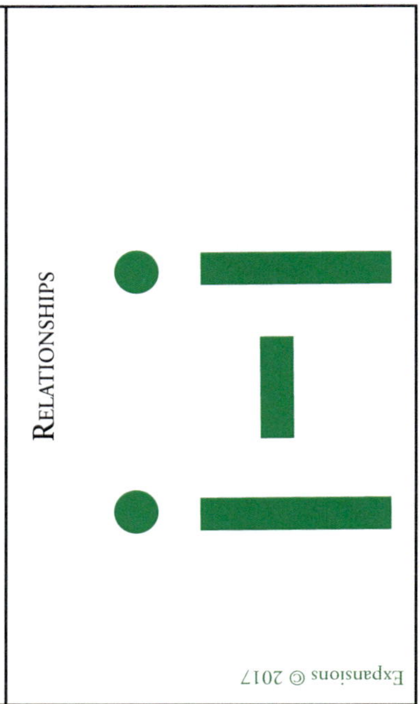
Relationships
Expansions © 2017

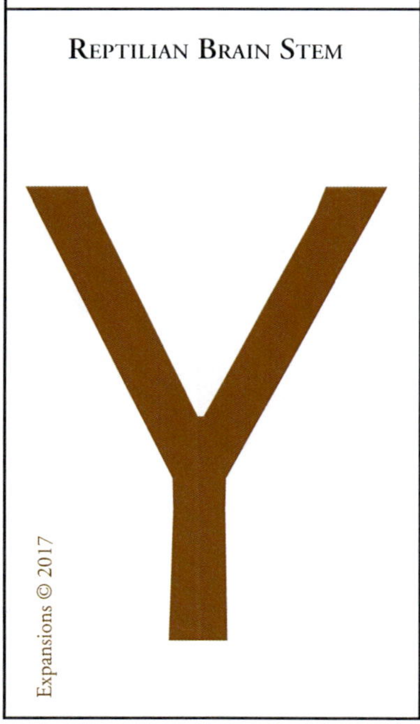
Reptilian Brain Stem
Expansions © 2017

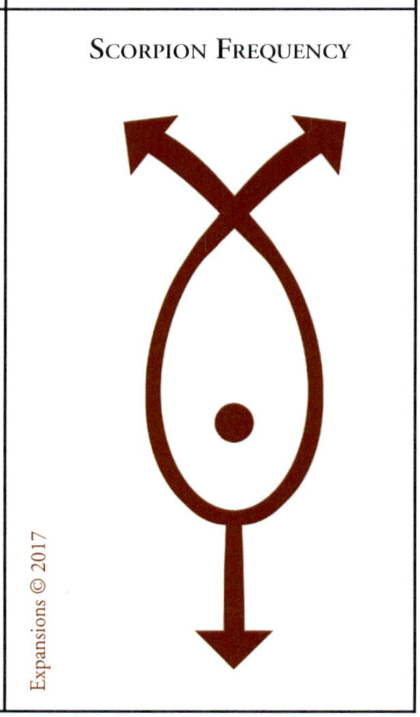
Scorpion Frequency
Expansions © 2017

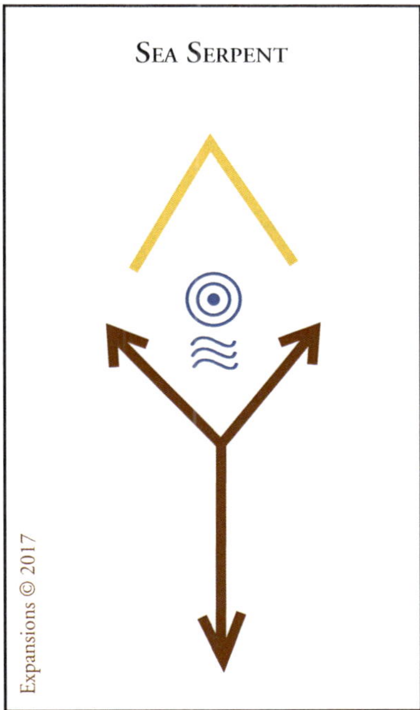
Sea Serpent
Expansions © 2017

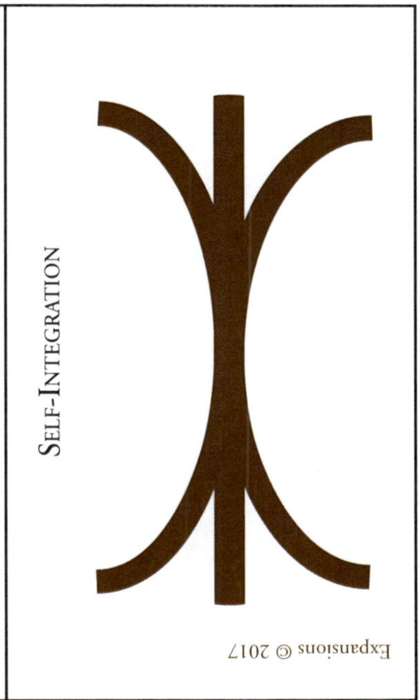
Self-Integration
Expansions © 2017

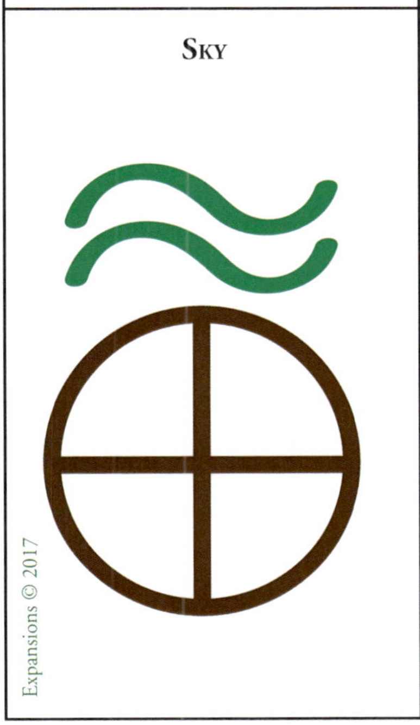
Sky
Expansions © 2017

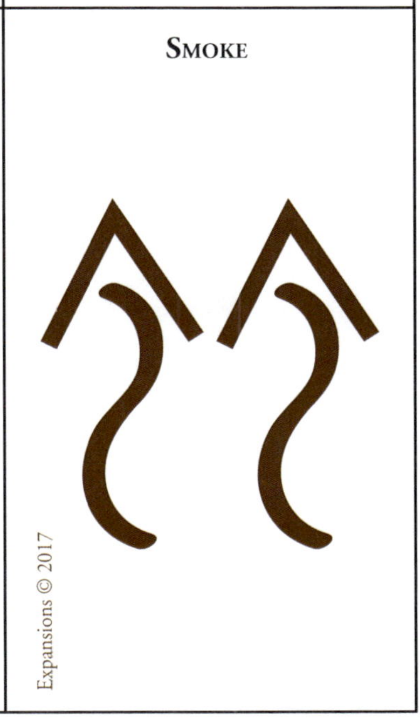
Smoke
Expansions © 2017

Spiritual & Intuition Connection
Expansions © 2017

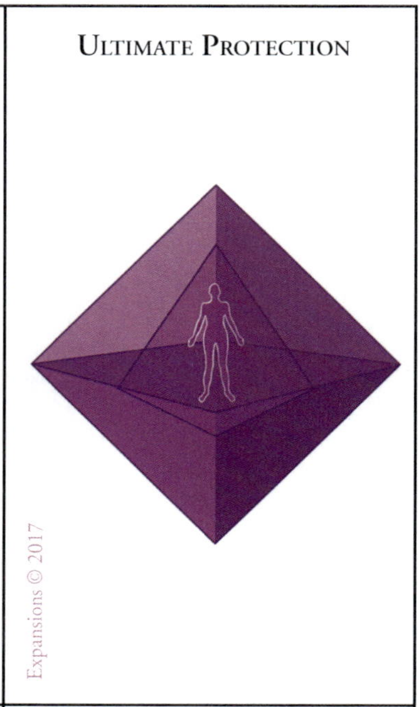
Ultimate Protection
Expansions © 2017

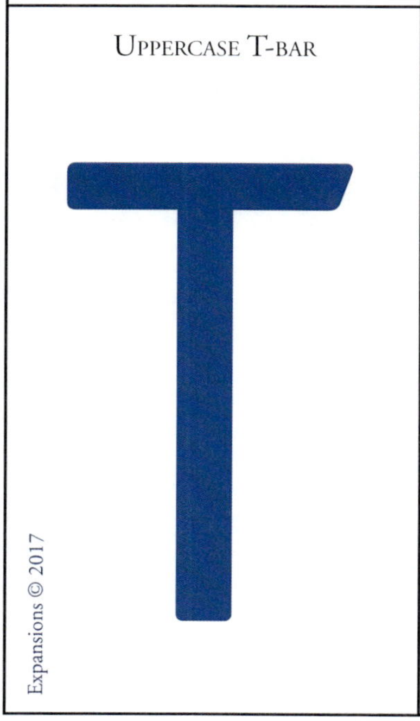
Uppercase T-bar
Expansions © 2017

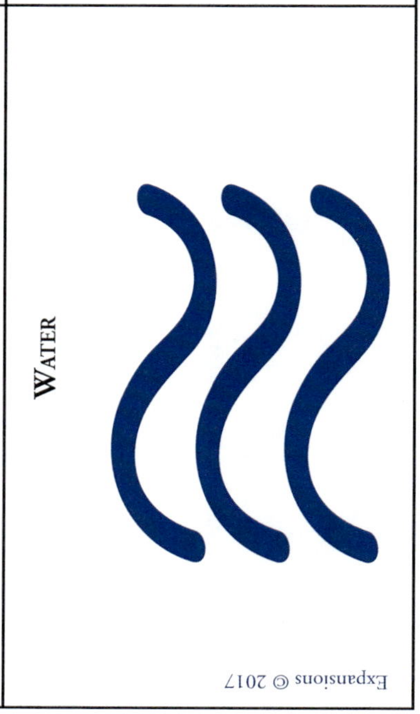
Water
Expansions © 2017

Wealth & Prosperity

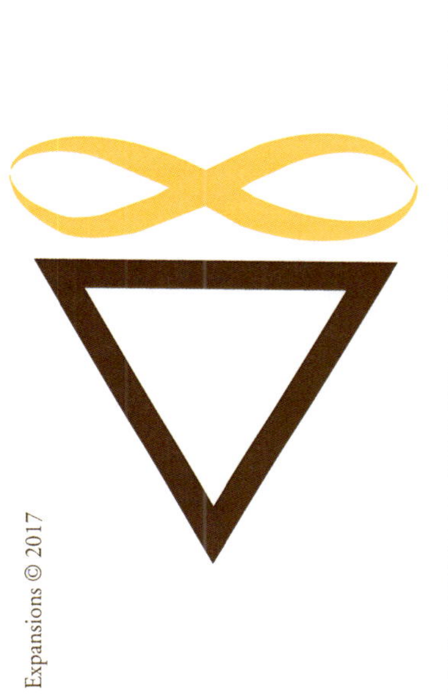

White Winged Dragon

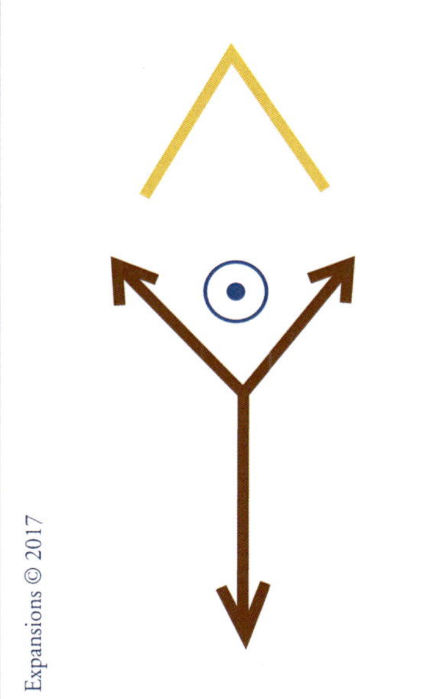

White Winged Dragon & White Winged Lion Merging

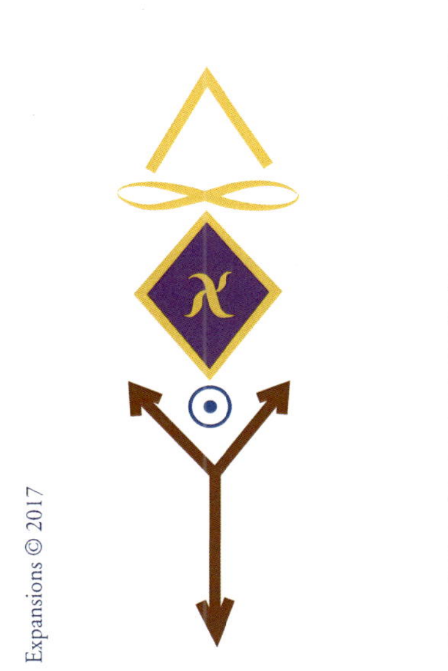

White Winged Lion

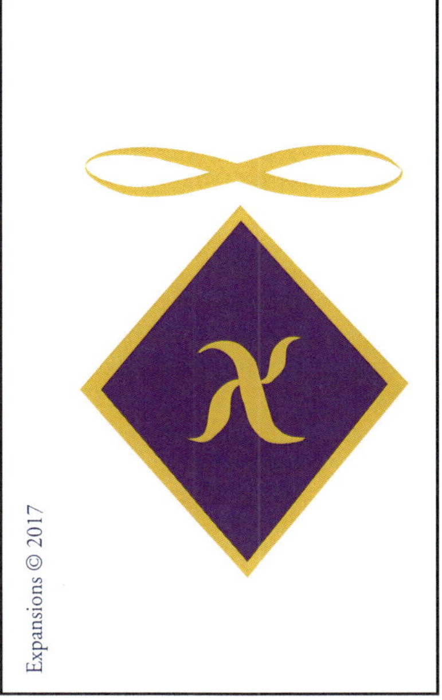

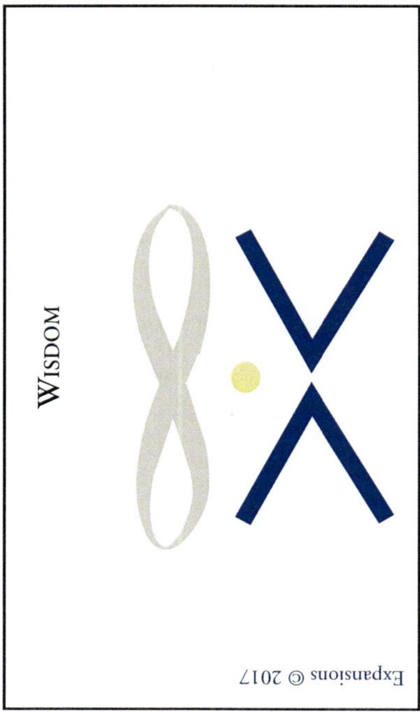
Wisdom
Expansions © 2017

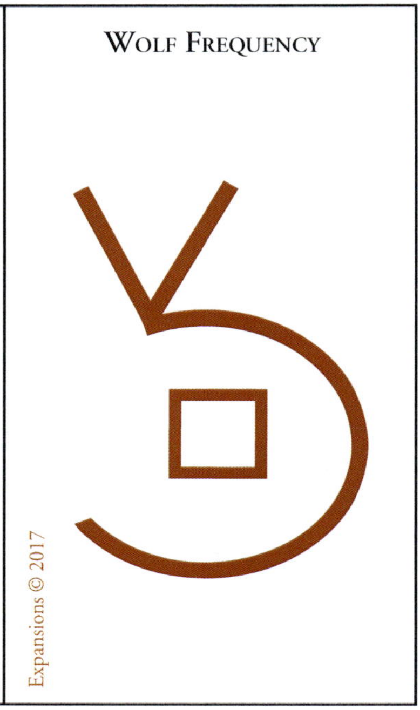
Wolf Frequency
Expansions © 2017

Glossary

A

Activation: When a program is brought to full function.

Affirmation: A statement that defines a course of action, or a state of inner being; repeating words many times by thinking, speaking, or writing it to bring new avenues of action into your conscious mind.

Animal Mind: Located at the solar plexus and controlled by the Reptilian brain stem; controls the physical body; in charge of fight or flight.

Aura: Your personal energy field.

Alien: A physical being from another planet.

Alter: Section or compartmentalized personality within a programming matrix.

Androgynous: Male and female combined without sexual distinction.

Archetype: Symbol or glyph from hyperspace or mind-patterns.

Astral Plane: The border zone between physical reality and hyperspace.

B

Bear Frequency Archetype: Increases protective nature; enhances introversion for self-study; best for males.

Bisexual: Sexually desiring both males and females.

Breasts Archetype: Enhances healthy breasts for Men and Women.

C

Cancellation Archetype: Removes anything unwanted.

Center: Your center is aligned along your spine, providing a safe space from which to work; you pull yourself into it by willing yourself into it.

Ceremony: Gathering to celebrate or honor an entity or Illuminati holiday.

Chakra Band: Energy center of the body and encompassing area.

Chakras: Along the human spinal column there are main nerve bundles called ganglions, which are esoterically called "chakras," a word that means "wheels" in Sanskrit. They form along the "S" curve of the spine, which looks like a snake. For this reason the chakra system is referred to as "Kundalini," the Sanskrit word for snake.

Collective Conscious Mind: The body of space that contains the accumulated known knowledge of humankind.

Collective Unconscious: The body of space that contains the accumulated thoughts of humankind; these established thought patterns directly affect what you move through today.

Communication Archetype: Speaking up as appropriate.

Conscious Mind: Contains your present.

Construct: Similar to a physical object created in the programming matrix to work with the alter in a specific function.

D

Deprogramming: Techniques to block and/or remove mind-control/programming.

Direct Awareness: To know by experiencing the knowledge.

DNA Sequences: This refers to the DNA sequences opening up in the body, which is a form of Kundalini activation. DNA codes are the instructions that tell your body what to do and be. Some instructions you are running at birth. These dictate that you will have blue eyes, two legs, two arms, etc. Others activate later in life, such as health conditions, ability to play music, sing, etc.

Dolphin Frequency Archetype: Eases mental shifting into hyperspace.

E

Emotional Balance Archetype: Obtains healthy emotional balance by balancing left and right hemispheres of the brain.

Energy: A physical substance consisting of shape, weight, consistency, and color.

ELF: Extra low frequency generally related to microwaves for mind-control purposes; energy.

ET (Extraterrestrial): Borderline physical/non-physical beings not bound to our reality.

Expansion Archetype: Increases and expands goals and desires.

F

Female Orgasm Archetype: Removes female frigidity; increase sexual responsiveness.

Frequency: A rate of vibration that distinguishes one flow of energy from all other flows.

G

God-Mind: Neutral energy; All That Is.

Golem: Human animal created from mud; animated by a controller.

Group-Mind: Formed when vibrations band together.

H

Habit Response: An established pattern of behavior that allows you to react to any given situation without thinking, whether physical or mental. It can be positive, negative, or neutral.

Happiness Archetype: Establishes happiness.

Horizontal Experience: Pulls you out into similar growth.

Hyperspace: A region of consciousness that exists outside of linear space and time.

I

Illuminati: Member or associate of one of the 13 ruling families on Earth.

Illusion: The way you perceive things to be.

Individualized Consciousness Archetype: Helps you rise out of the Group-Mind into Your Own connection with Mind and Personal yourOversoul and God-Mind.

K

Know by Knowing: To understand through direct awareness; to understand the feeling of an experience.

Knowledge: Information.

L

Language of Hyperspace: The Original Language that emanates from the Mind of God consisting of color, tone, and archetype (symbol).

Leadership Archetype: installs Self-Leadership.

Lion Frequency Archetype: Increases your direct awareness to God-Mind power.

Logos Christos Archetype: Healing generator on specific body locations.

Love: Neutral energy that emanates from God-Mind that does not discriminate.

Lyrae: Star system in the Milky Way Galaxy that is the origin point for all humans.

M

Macrocosm: God-Mind; All That Is; the larger picture of everything.

Male Orgasm Archetype: Removes impotence; increases virility.

Matrix, Programming: The structure in the mind that facilitates mind-control; 13 x 13 x 13, which equals 2,197 compartments.

Meditation: A process that moves you beyond words and connects you with silence, the level of feeling; the listening from which information is gathered; centered in the right brain.

Mental Balance Archetype: Creates mental balance in all areas.

Merging with Aspects of Alternative Selves Archetype: Bring current goals to fruition by merging with your Self in the Eternal Now.

Microcosm: You; a world in miniature.

Mind-Pattern: Blueprint of a persons' thoughts.

N

Negative: Negative is not "bad," but merely a condition that exists; the opposite of positive, which explains another part of the same experience.

New Beginnings Archetype: Start new projects, relationships, health, finances.

New World Religion: Global religion.

New World Order (NWO): Global government dictatorship being created by the Illuminati.

O

Objective Listening: Listening and evaluating without judgment or criticism.

Objective Observing: Watching and evaluating without judgment or criticism.

Overall Healing Archetype: Heals body, mind, and soul.

Oversoul: Neutral energy that comes out of God-Mind; your

Oversoul is to you what your Earth parents are to your body. Your Oversoul is your point of origin out of God-Mind.

Oversoul Archetype: Your Point of Origin out of the God-Mind.

P

Pineal Gland: Organ at the center of the head.

Positive: Positive is not better than negative, but is merely a condition that exists; the opposite of negative, which explains another part of the same experience.

Power Archetype: Increases personal power via your mental abilities.

Prayer: Request that affects the results of meditation; centered in the left-brain.

Pregnancy Archetype: Increases fertility; maintain healthy pregnancy.

Pregnancy Prevention Archetype: Cancels your fertility.

Proactive Learning: Active learning; gathering knowledge before an experience occurs.

Psychic Energy: Your personal energy; it flows back and forth, and is horizontal.

R

Reactive Learning: Passive learning; gathering knowledge after an experience occurs.

Reality: The way things really are; it may vary considerably from your perception of the way you think things are.

Rejuvenation Archetype: Enhances physical, mental, emotional, spiritual rejuvenation.

Release & Resolve Past Issues Archetype: Cleans out what you no longer need.

Relationships Archetype: Improves and enhances people connection.

Reptilian: A being with lizard-like characteristics from either the inner Earth or Draco star system; colonized Lemuria.

S

Self-Integration Archetype: Brown Merger Archetype; merges all parts of Self into one; great deprogramming aid.

Shapeshifter: A person who physically changes from one species to another.

Silence: The deepest level of inner awareness; the level of feeling; you connect with your Oversoul and God-Mind within silence.

Simultaneous Existence: All lifelines occurring at the same moment in the Eternal Now.

Spirituality: A state of inner being.

Spiritual & Intuition Connection Archetype: Improves conscious connection with your Oversoul and God-Mind.

Soul-Personality: Individual strand of an Oversoul.

Subconscious Mind: Contains your memories, moment-by-moment, lifeline-by-lifeline.

Sub-Personality: A group of similar emotions that becomes strong enough to develop its own consciousness; a sub-personality is not you, but it is a part of you.

Superconscious Mind: Provides the direct link to your Oversoul and God-Mind.

T

T-Bar: Archetype emanating from the pineal gland relating to balance.

Trigger: Sensory input that opens a program.

U

Ultimate Protection Archetype: Protects whatever you desire.

Universal Energy: Energy that is available to everyone; using it allows you to keep your psychic energy; it flows up and down, and is vertical.

Universal Law: Rules and regulations that pervade all creation; emanates from God-Mind.

V

Vertical Experience: Pulls you up into new growth.

Vibration: Frequency rate of an energy.

Vibratory Imprint: Accumulated feelings of like experiences; they cause you to react to your experiences of today through your accumulated feelings of yesterday.

Visualization: Creating a mental scenario that can be manifested either mentally or physically; centered at the pineal gland.

W

Wealth & Prosperity Archetype: Increases finances.

Wisdom: Knowledge applied.

Wisdom Archetype: Enhances your correct use of knowledge.

Wolf Frequency Archetype: Enhances family relationships.

Y

You: Individualized neutral energy.

Index

C

D

E

F

V

W

Y

Testimonials

"My daily use of archetypes makes my life complete. I start every day with the Protection Archetype. Using archetypes this past year helped facilitate a New Beginning filled with Happiness and Abundance. These archetypes truly enhanced my life!"

—Lorraine S., New York

"Using the archetypes is now an effortless daily practice that offers me a tranquil approach to my many obstacles, allowing my inner desires to become reality. I thank Stewart and Janet daily for the way their work changed my life. I am learning to think differently with positive results!"

—Karen D., Australia

"The Protection Archetype works in a practical and almost unbelievable way. One day, it helped me find the expensive electronic key pad that I use in my real estate business. After losing it, the thought came to look on top of my car—it was still there even though I had traveled back and forth through the city, including several stoplights along the way. Nothing is by chance, and I know that I was being Protected!"

—Randy A., St. Louis, MO

"Archetypes are like powerful energetic keys that I use daily, just like I use my car and house keys. My eternal thanks to the Swerdlows for making these tools available for everyone!"

—Ximena P., New Zealand

"Stewart and Janet's archetypes are an invaluable aid. In the areas of Happiness and Protection, they have proved themselves to us time and time again. We are now using the New Beginnings Archetype, so our bags are packed and we are looking forward to a brighter future! Thank you, Stewart and Janet."

—Phil & Claire D., United Kingdom

"I know several mental and physical healthcare professionals who already use these archetypes. I think that these archetypes someday will be regularly incorporated into the psychological and medical fields. My personal experience with them has been phenomenal!"

—Shannon S., California